Functional Core for Women

Targeted Training for Glutes and Abs

Kia Williams

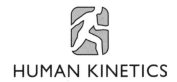

HUMAN KINETICS

Library of Congress Cataloging-in-Publication Data

Names: Williams, Kia, 1988- author.
Title: Functional core for women : targeted training for glutes and abs /
  Kia Williams.
Description: First edition. | Champaign, IL : Human Kinetics, [2024] |
  Includes bibliographical references.
Identifiers: LCCN 2022048280 (print) | LCCN 2022048281 (ebook) | ISBN
  9781718211582 (paperback) | ISBN 9781718211599 (epub) | ISBN
  9781718211605 (pdf)
Subjects: LCSH: Abdominal exercises. | Buttocks exercises. | Exercise for
  women. | BISAC: HEALTH & FITNESS / Exercise / General | HEALTH & FITNESS
  / Women's Health
Classification: LCC GV508 W55 2024 (print) | LCC GV508 (ebook) | DDC
  613.7/1--dc23/eng/20221026
LC record available at https://lccn.loc.gov/2022048280
LC ebook record available at https://lccn.loc.gov/2022048281

ISBN: 978-1-7182-1158-2 (print)

Senior Acquisitions Editor: Michelle Earle; **Developmental Editor:** Amy Stahl; **Managing Editor:** Hannah Werner; **Copyeditor:** Joanna Hatzopoulos Portman; **Graphic Designer:** Denise Lowry; **Cover Designer:** Keri Evans; **Cover Design Specialist:** Susan Rothermel Allen; **Photographs (cover):** Texture, Tuomas A. Lehtinen /Moment/Getty Images; Photo © Human Kinetics; **Photographs (interior):** © Human Kinetics; **Photo Asset Manager:** Laura Fitch; **Photo Production Specialist:** Amy M. Rose; **Photo Production Manager:** Jason Allen; **Senior Art Manager:** Kelly Hendren; **Illustrations:** Heidi Richter/© Human Kinetics; **Printer:** Versa Press

Human Kinetics books are available at special discounts for bulk purchase. Special editions or book excerpts can also be created to specification. For details, contact the Special Sales Manager at Human Kinetics.

Printed in the United States of America   10 9 8 7 6 5 4 3 2 1

The paper in this book is certified under a sustainable forestry program.

Human Kinetics
1607 N. Market Street
Champaign, IL 61820
USA

United States and International
Website: **US.HumanKinetics.com**
Email: info@hkusa.com
Phone: 1-800-747-4457

Canada
Website: **Canada.HumanKinetics.com**
Email: info@hkcanada.com

E8531

This work is dedicated to anyone
who allows themselves to be malleable and open
to learning something different from someone different.

CONTENTS

EXERCISE FINDER

Chapter 7 Warm-Up and Activation Exercises

Core Activation

Chapter 8 Stretches

Stretches for the Core

ACKNOWLEDGMENTS

Thank you to the wonderful team at Human Kinetics who contributed to making this book a reality. I express great gratitude to senior acquisitions editor Michelle Earle, who has trusted, supported, and amplified my vision and voice in many aspects of fitness and movement. Much appreciation is extended to developmental editor Amy Stahl for intently working alongside me on this book and bringing authentic connections across the pages.

Finally, to the most important people who have known me the longest—my parents and my sisters: Thank you for your unwavering support, advocacy, and unconditional love. Your cheerleading and championing of me throughout my writing journey have kept this project alive. Thank you for your encouragement and belief in the process and in me. We make a great team. I love you.

INTRODUCTION

Sedentary lifestyles and preventable diseases are on the rise. Also on the rise are common exercise injuries stemming from lack of movement, improper movement, weak core muscles, and lack of knowledge of the core's true function. Another concern is the scarcity of credible information to help mitigate these issues. Most exercise books that focus on core muscles discuss only sculpting, toning, and the aesthetics of the abdominal muscles (abs). They neglect to expand on and emphasize the importance of the entire core—which includes the gluteal muscles (glutes)—working in synergy for optimal exercise performance, injury reduction, and improved quality of life. *Functional Core for Women: Targeted Training for Glutes and Abs* examines the function of the collective core muscles as well as the lifestyle benefits of having a strong core.

Strengthening the core can improve athletic performance; reduce risk of injuries, aches, and pains; and improve balance and mobility. This book focuses on the two primary anatomical regions (abs and glutes) that make up the core and aid in life's daily functions. It delivers a collection of 49 of the best individual exercises for the abs and glutes along with 24 exercises for warm-up and activation and stretches, and 6 quick exercise routines with multiple sequences for strengthening your muscular assets. These exercises are functional and adaptable. They are easy to do with or without equipment and in nearly any location.

Despite the clear health benefits of core strengthening, popular culture promotes the myth that fitness and quality health are based on appearance, such as looking slim, sculpted, muscular, or toned. Some people are born with these looks but may not have the health benefits of a strong core. In addition, while you can achieve changes in appearance through training (e.g., training the glutes in specific ways that affect size or shape), relying on aesthetics is not an accurate way to measure health and fitness. Unfortunately, convincing people of the facts and debunking this myth can be difficult since misinformation spreads quickly and is unregulated online and in other media channels. Rather than perpetuating or falling into fads and inaccurate exercise information, the information in this book is based on sound research to help you achieve your personal goals for your core, whether your goals are for better health, improved functional movement, or to improve your core's physical appearance. This book is written with women in mind, since women are often subjected to media and cultural influence and scrutiny of their appearance.

This book is written to inform and empower women through safe and realistic exercise.

This book guides you through the process of understanding and training your core. It defines and explains specific core muscles, clarifies their purpose, and describes their function. It offers exercises that target the abs and glutes and will help you to move functionally and safely. In addition, the book shows you how to tie together various exercises into specific training protocols and programs while keeping exercise simple, versatile, and fun.

This book's unique, detailed approach to working your abs and glutes will help you do the following:

- Establish core strength.
- Cultivate body awareness, control, and balance.
- Reduce vulnerability to injury.
- Improve your overall fitness.
- Understand the function and purpose of core muscles.
- Challenge your existing fitness level.
- Change the way your body looks and feels.

In addition, this exercise guide will help you do the following:

- Debunk myths and misconceptions about the abs and glutes.
- Learn fresh exercise tips for targeting and training your abs and glutes.
- Follow step-by-step cues on how to safely and optimally perform core-focused exercises.
- Learn ways to improve the physical appearance of your abs and glutes through exercise.

This book invites you to discover and explore scientifically backed research coupled with a fresh catalog of core exercises that will deliver optimal benefits and results. Enjoy the journey!

PART I

UNDERSTANDING THE CORE

CHAPTER 1

Core = Abs + Glutes

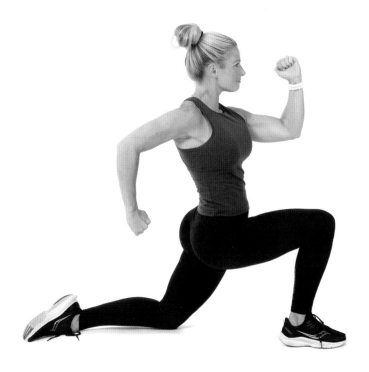

The core is the center of the body. Contrary to popular misconceptions, the core does not consist only of six-pack abs; it comprises all the muscles attached to the pelvis and spine and that make up the front, back, and sides of the torso. The core includes muscles that stabilize the hips and shoulders while the arms and legs functionally move, such as muscles of the chest, the back, and the entire abdominal wall, to name a few. As an added bonus, the glutes assist movements of the pelvis, hips, and torso, so they are considered minor core muscles as well. To understand the core, you need to know how all these muscles work together as a unit.

This chapter discusses the structure and basic function of the abdominal and gluteal muscles to help you understand the core muscles and the exercises in this book.

When discussing fitness performance, the term *muscular strength* refers to the relative measurement of the amount of force you can exert or the amount of weight you can lift. *Muscular endurance* is the ability of your muscles to remain active for an extended period of time before failure or exhaustion. *Hypertrophy* is the increase in muscular development and size. Refer to chapter 3 for more details on these three topics.

Anatomy of the Abdominal Muscles

Abdominal muscles (abs) are located in the front of the body (anteriorly) between the ribs and pelvis. These muscles work to support, stabilize, and protect the torso and vertebral column, allow movement, and hold organs in place. The four main abdominal muscles emphasized for exercise purposes are the transverse abdominis, rectus abdominis, external obliques, and internal obliques (see figure 1.1).

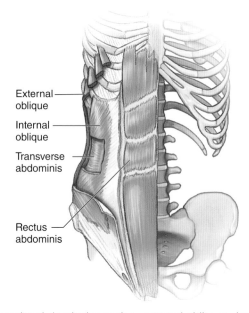

FIGURE 1.1   Four anterior abdominal muscles: external obliques, internal obliques, transverse abdominis, and rectus abdominis.

To help you train more efficiently and reach your fitness goals more effectively, this book distinguishes between inner and outer abdominal muscles. The well-developed muscles that you would like to see in the mirror require exercising and strengthening the inner muscles that can't be seen with the naked eye. To achieve strong, sculpted abs, you need the inner and outer abdominal muscles to work together.

The outer abdominal muscles include the rectus abdominis (so-called six-pack abs), external obliques, internal obliques, and erector spinae. Although the erector spinae muscles are actually back muscles that run from the base of the skull all the way down to the pelvis, they are considered part of the abdominal muscle group; they work with other abdominal (and glute) muscles to stabilize the torso. The inner abdominal muscles include the transverse abdominis, internal obliques, and multifidus. Multifidus muscles are located deep in the back, on either side of the spine, from the cervical spine all the way down to the lumbar spine (see figure 1.2).

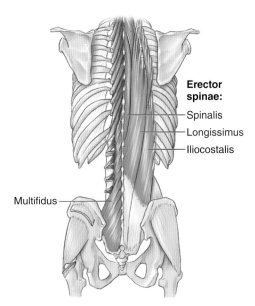

FIGURE 1.2   Intermediate and deep muscle layers of the spine, including the erector spinae and multifidus, which are also considered part of the abdominal group.

The rectus abdominis is a pair of long muscles that run vertically along the front of the abdomen. Its function is to move the rib cage and pelvis, compress internal organs, and provide tension to the abdominal wall. Misinformation about how six-packs are developed has led exercisers to overtrain this muscle group to achieve the look of six-pack abs. Everyone has a six-pack, but some are less pronounced than others. There are a cluster of factors that help unveil the sculpted six-pack abs, such as good nutrition, resistance training, and cardiorespiratory exercise. To clarify myths and misconceptions, everyone has anatomical six-pack abs and suggested exercises in this book will help to strengthen all core muscles for better functional performance.

External obliques are the outermost abdominal muscles. Located on each side of the rectus abdominis, they make up the side (lateral) part of the abdominal wall. They each function on one side of the body (unilaterally) to allow twisting (rotation) of the torso as well as side bending (lateral flexion and extension). Lateral flexion and extension are the actions of bending side to side.

Internal oblique muscles are a thin muscle layer of the lateral abdominal wall that is situated toward the front (anteriorly) on the sides of the abdomen. They function as an accessory muscle of breathing, aid lateral flexion of the torso, and act in opposition to the external obliques (contralaterally) during rotation. In other words, if you twist to the right, the right-side internal obliques contract while the left-side external obliques contract. In addition, internal obliques can function together at the same time (bilaterally).

The transverse abdominis is one of the innermost abdominal muscles, and it wraps around the torso trunk from front to back. Its function is to maintain abdominal wall tension to support the torso, stabilize the lumbar spine and pelvis before the limbs move, and protect the internal organs. Proper activation of the transverse abdominis can help to alleviate back pain.

Core Training Myths

You have likely heard or read all kinds of advice about how to train your core. Some of that advice may be good; some is not so good. Let's separate myths from facts regarding some of the things people say on this topic.

Myth 1: The Core Is the Same as the Abs

Fact: The abs are just one piece of the pie (or core). The core is made up of multiple muscle groups (e.g., the diaphragm, transverse abdominis, erector spinae, and multifidus) that work together to support and protect the pelvis, hips, and spine. Abs do not work alone in core function; back and glute muscles are involved in core work as well. (Glutes are discussed in more detail in the next section.)

Myth 2: A Chiseled Six-Pack Equates to a Strong Core

Fact: While a six-pack may be considered attractive by some standards, it does not mean that someone with a visible six-pack can out-plank someone whose six-pack isn't as pronounced. Every person has six-pack abs as part of their anatomy (the rectus abdominis), but true core strength involves more muscular engagement, not just the rectus abdominis.

Myth 3: Doing More Crunches Will Build Abs

Fact: Your abdominal muscles already exist, so you don't have much building to do; when training the abs, you are not erecting a building from the ground up. Also, all muscles of the body need recovery time after targeting exercise work. During the recovery phase of exercise, muscles get stronger and more developed. Depriving the muscles of this recovery time leads to overtraining, which results in weakened muscles, injury, and loss of stability—everything you *don't* want. The abs are active during most of your functional, daily movement patterns, so they work without you even thinking about it. In addition, crunches are not the only way to chisel your abs. Some fitness professionals argue that crunches are not the most beneficial way to build your abs because they are not functional movements, and the repetitive forward flexion of the spine could cause unnecessary compression on spinal discs.

Anatomy of the Gluteal Muscles

Gluteal muscles (glutes) are the largest and strongest muscles of the body. The gluteal region (also called buttocks or butt) comprises a group of three superficial muscles: gluteus maximus, gluteus medius, and gluteus minimus (figure 1.3). These three muscle groupings originate from the ilium, sacrum, and coccyx, and they insert on the femur (covered by muscles in figure 1.3). They mainly act to abduct and extend the lower limb at the hip joint and assist in moving and stabilizing the pelvis, hips, and torso. (*Abduct* means to move a limb away from the midline of the body; *extend* means to increase the angle at a joint.)

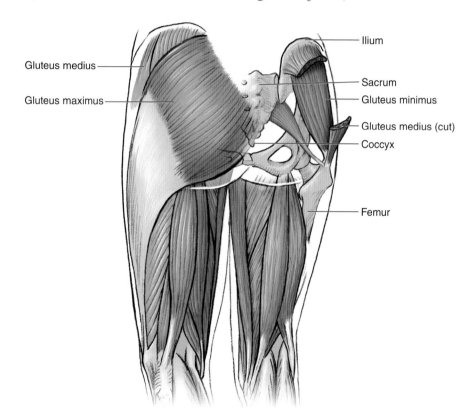

FIGURE 1.3   Gluteal region.

Gluteus maximus (glute max) is the largest of the glute muscles, and it produces the shape of the butt. The glute max extends and laterally rotates the femur (thigh bone) at the hip joint, and it is used for forward movement such as stepping up, running, and climbing. The upper fibers can abduct and the lower fibers can adduct the lower limb or femur and the hip. The glute max plays a role in stabilizing and balancing the pelvis and maintaining an upright posture.

The fan-shaped gluteus medius (glute medius) takes up less space on your butt than the glute max, and it lies between the glute max and gluteus minimus. Located on the lateral region of the upper buttocks, it is the primary mover of abduction at the hip joint and assists in external and internal rotation at the hip joint. Glute medius is an important muscle for maintaining stability of the pelvis when performing lateral movement patterns.

Butt-Busting Myths About the Glutes

There's a lot of misinformation about how to train your glutes to get the performance or appearance that you want from these muscles. What's true, and what's not? Let's set the record straight on three common misbeliefs.

Myth 1: Do Squats to Grow Your Butt

Fact: The squat is a great exercise to help increase strength in the muscles of your lower half, but it is not the most effective glute-building exercise. Glute building works better when combining the squat with other exercises such as the deadlift, hip bridge, and hip abduction. Squats help strengthen your glutes, which can result in the appearance of definition, lift, fullness, and roundness of your butt. Genetics actually plays a big role in the shape and size of your butt. If it does not run in your family, then it will be a harder gain for you. The silver lining is that since the glutes are muscles, muscle hypertrophy is possible. However, you have to lift heavy weights and tax the gluteal muscle fibers to accomplish that kind of muscle growth.

Myth 2: You Can Fake It

Fact: For photographic purposes, you can practice poking your booty up and out (anterior pelvic tilt), crunch in your lower back, step one leg forward, and put a crease in your hip to have an appearance of a rounder and bigger butt. But not only is that posture a lot of work, the compression on your lower back is painful. Once the picture is taken and posted online, what will be your explanation for the not-so-plump butt in real life? It is a temporary, superficial fix. Another way to fake it is through surgery, which comes at a high price to your wallet and your health. Butt augmentations come with life-threatening risks that may not be worth the gamble.

Myth 3: Increasing Calories to Increase the Size of a Specific Body Part Is the Answer

Fact: There is no such thing as spot gain. In general, increased caloric intake in excess of what the body burns will result in overall weight gain. It is impossible to signal to the food being consumed and digested to store itself as fat in specified areas. Your best chance at changing the shape of your butt is through balanced nutrition coupled with purposeful exercise.

Gluteus minimus (glute min) is the smallest and deepest of the three gluteal muscles. It is similar in structure and function to the glute medius. It is located deep in the posterior hip region and under the glute medius. The main function of the glute min is abduction and lateral rotation at the hip joint. The glute min is important for securing the pelvis and preventing it from dropping to one side of the body when the body is in motion.

Now that you have a better understanding of how the core works as a whole unit with anatomical purpose and function, you can better comprehend how and why core training is beneficial. This understanding also sets you up for success in core exercise selection and performance.

CHAPTER 2

Core Functions and Mechanics

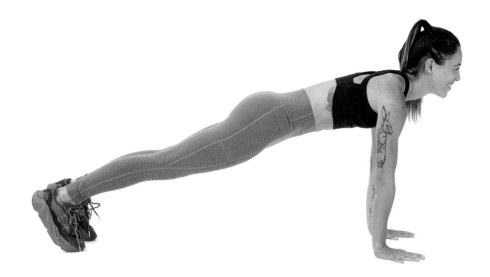

The core is important for life endurance (or life longevity), for distributing load to support and protect the spine, and for absorbing and transferring force between the lower and upper body. "Core training, abdominal training, and core stiffness and stability are all essential components for pain control, performance enhancement, and injury resilience" (McGill 2016, p. 154). Core training is the conditioning of the stabilizing muscles of the abdomen, back, and pelvic regions. Proper core training can support the combined function of your core muscle groups.

Injury to the spine typically occurs as a result of improper biomechanics and movement patterns. A strong and conditioned core forms a 360-degree armor of protection for the spine. This armor supports, stabilizes, and protects the spine and pelvis from injury during exercise performance, multiplanar movement patterns, and common everyday slips, trips, and falls.

Core Functioning

The abdominal muscles function to support your torso. They maintain balance, strength, and posture to keep you upright while standing and comfortable while lying down. The abs directly support the weight of the upper body for alignment and stability, and they protect important bones and joints such as the spine, pelvis, and shoulders from injury and vulnerability to life's wear and tear. The abs form the central support system that aids in the entire body moving functionally and with purpose, which also leads to better balance and stability. Your abs help move your pelvis, thighs, spine, head, and neck, which means they are active even when you walk. In addition, the abs connect to the shoulders and the hips. Essentially, without strong, functioning abs, the arms and legs would have a tough time moving with purpose and intention. Strong abs go a long way in helping you stand upright, walk efficiently, run faster, kick higher, and have better physical performance.

The abs also function as a protective barrier for your organs. They help to protect soft internal tissues in the event of a fall or impact. They also assist in breathing and holding your organs in place by enveloping the organs like a corset, compressing them, and sending a message to them to function in synchrony when you breathe, move, cough, sneeze, laugh, urinate, and defecate. Strong abs support better breathing and digestive health. They also assist in moving things out of the body, such as when vomiting, defecating, urinating, and giving birth.

Strong abs have practical purpose in your daily life. Improving the strength and function of the abs improves posture, balance, athletic performance, confidence, and mood. All these functional benefits can also improve the way you look and feel. Figure 2.1 summarizes the benefits of training the abs.

The gluteal muscles function to do the following:

- Keep the body upright.
- Move the body forward.
- Maintain proper pelvic alignment.
- Support the lower back during lifting.
- Assist with balance.

The glutes are responsible for hip extension (to increase the angle at the hip joint), internal hip rotation (turning your thigh bone inward), and hip abduction (taking the leg away from the midline of the body). These functional bodily movements are responsible for standing; skipping; running; bending over; getting up from a seated or lying position; stepping up; walking; jumping, twisting, and turning; and simply moving your body in multiple planes of motion or directions. The glutes attach to muscles in the hips and back, so much like the function of the abs, the glutes support your body weight, alignment, and stability, and they help keep you upright. Strong glutes keep the pelvis aligned and posture ideal for performing various daily activities and exercises. Strong, functioning

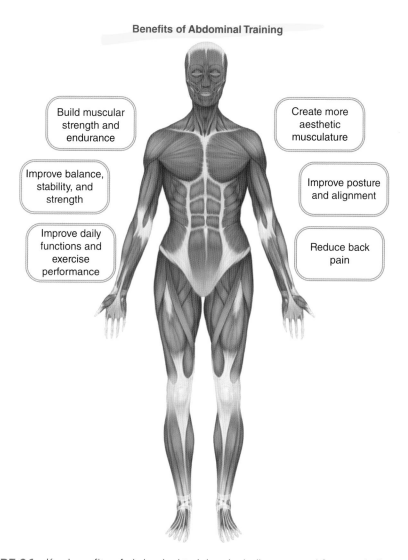

Benefits of Abdominal Training

Build muscular strength and endurance

Create more aesthetic musculature

Improve balance, stability, and strength

Improve posture and alignment

Improve daily functions and exercise performance

Reduce back pain

FIGURE 2.1 Key benefits of abdominal training, including postural form and alignment.

glutes will help the hip joints move more efficiently and respond better to quick, dynamic movements (e.g., a quick change in direction) and powerful movements (e.g., kicks, jumps, and pushes). Strong glutes will help improve overall bodily stability, strength, power, and movement. Depending on how you train them, they can also change the physical shape of your butt in a way that could make it more aesthetically appealing to your personal standards. Figure 2.2 summarizes the benefits of training the glutes.

Research indicates that contraction of the deep abdominal muscles may assist or help stimulate the contraction of the gluteus maximus to aid in control of anterior pelvic rotation (Kim and Kim 2015). To better

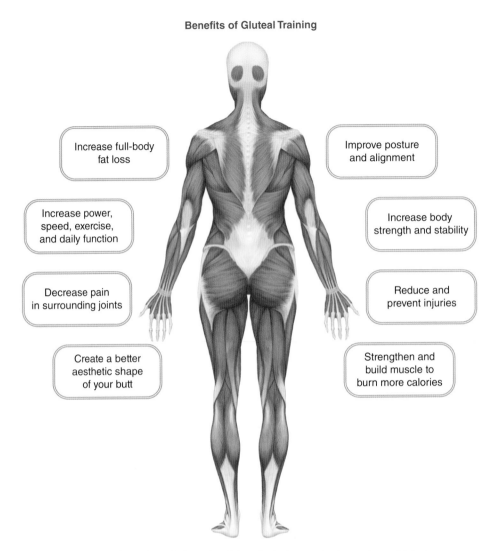

Benefits of Gluteal Training

Increase full-body
fat loss

Improve posture
and alignment

Increase power,
speed, exercise,
and daily function

Increase body
strength and stability

Decrease pain
in surrounding joints

Reduce and
prevent injuries

Create a better
aesthetic shape
of your butt

Strengthen and
build muscle to
burn more calories

FIGURE 2.2 Key benefits of gluteal training, including reducing pain and injuries.

understand this connection, stand up and brace your abdominal muscles
to set your posture strong. Notice that your glutes and pelvic floor probably engaged as well. Now bend your knees and turn your body to one
side. One of your hips went farther forward than the other. That action
is an anterior pelvic rotation. You perform this movement when you do
exercises with spinal rotation, such as windshield wiper, sumo crossbody
reach, and sumo squat twist (see Exercise Finder). For this type of movement to be possible, the transverse abdominis assist or help stimulate the
contraction of the gluteus maximus while the gluteus maximus sends a
message to the pelvis to align and shift. In other words, the core works
as a whole, integrated unit.

Core Training Mechanics

For successful core training and injury prevention, it is best to mentally prepare before moving your body in an exercise. When training your core, make sure you know what to expect for the movement pattern, the purpose of the exercise, how your body should look and feel from start to finish of each repetition of the exercise (optimal form and alignment), and how to safely get into and out of each exercise.

Be mindful of your posture (form and alignment) in all exercises. Most often, whether you are standing, seated, or lying on the floor (see figure 2.3), optimal posture is to have the ears aligned with the shoulders, the spine long, the shoulders aligned with the hips, and the hips aligned with the heels. The shoulders should remain relaxed while you breathe deeply.

Keep breathing throughout the exercise. A rule of thumb is to forcefully exhale on the effort or what feels like the more challenging phase of each repetition of the exercise and inhale on what feels like the less taxing phase. For example, in a squat, inhale as you bend your knees and lower your hips down toward the earth, and exhale as you resist the earth and rise up to a standing position.

Never hold your breath, suck in your stomach, or forcefully pull the navel toward the spine (called *imprinting*); these actions inhibit functional movement, increase instability in the spine, and impair the integrity of all movement patterns. Instead, bracing is encouraged.

Dr. Stuart McGill, a professor of spinal biomechanics, developed a technique called abdominal bracing. Bracing is about fine-tuning and stiffening the muscles of the abdominal wall and controlling positions for proper core stability to help prevent injury and maintain integrity of the spine. Ikeda and McGill (2012) state, "We prefer teaching bracing to encourage activation of all components of the abdominal wall; this immediately reduces pain in many patients" (p. 163). For optimal effect, you brace before moving.

How do you brace? The terms *bracing*, *engaging*, and *activating* will show up often in this book when referring to muscle contraction and stiffness. Essentially, these terms encourage an understanding in the mind that communicates voluntary muscular contraction to the body. Mostly these words refer to stabilizing the spine and having optimal muscle activation before, during, and after performing an exercise. To know if you are bracing properly, put your hands on your waist with the palms over the ribs and fingertips to the sides of the navel. Push the fingertips into the belly. On an exhalation, stiffen (brace) your abdominal wall; if you are bracing properly, you will feel your stiffened muscles push against your fingers (see figure 2.4). Your muscles should feel like they are a girdle of support to your torso.

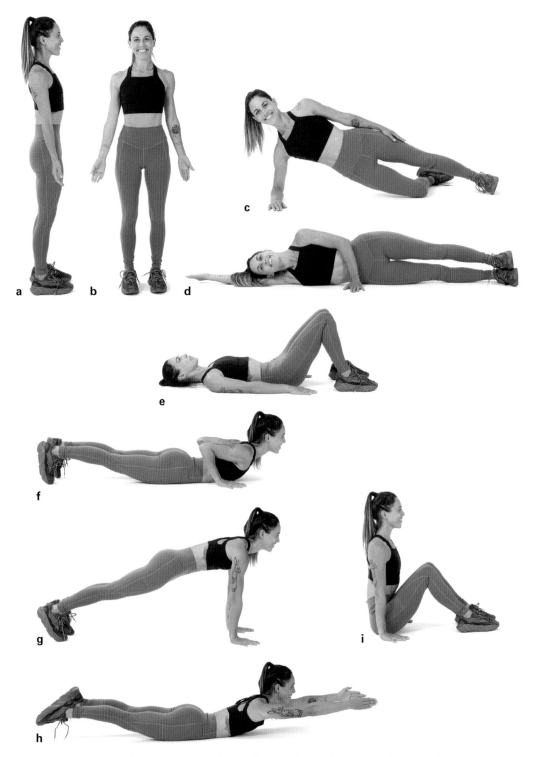

FIGURE 2.3   Body alignment: (*a-b*) Standing—side and front view; (*c-d*) side lying—on forearm and on side with bottom arm extended; (*e*) supine; (*f-h*) prone—with palms on floor, in plank position, and in Superman position; and (*i*) seated.

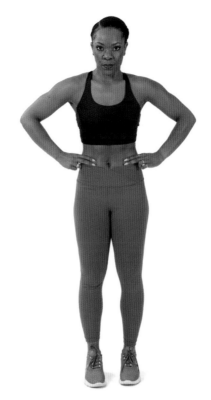

FIGURE 2.4   Optimal bracing form.

Caution: Weakness, Loss of Function, and Injury

A sedentary lifestyle of prolonged daily sitting deactivates the glutes, and poor posture inhibits the abs from working effectively.

If you don't use them, you lose them.

It is recommended that every 60 minutes that you are awake, you stand up with good posture and do movements that move your body from side to side, front to back, and twist and turn to target the core muscles; focus especially on the abs and glutes with exercises provided in this book. Injuries such as muscle strains can occur from overstretching and overuse. Regular warming up prior to exercise, proper exercise technique, and cooling down and stretching help prevent exercise-related injuries.

Better understanding of the function of core muscles helps to inform training decisions based on desires, needs, physical abilities, and personal goals.

PART II

PLANNING FOR RESULTS

CHAPTER 3
Identifying Personal Goals

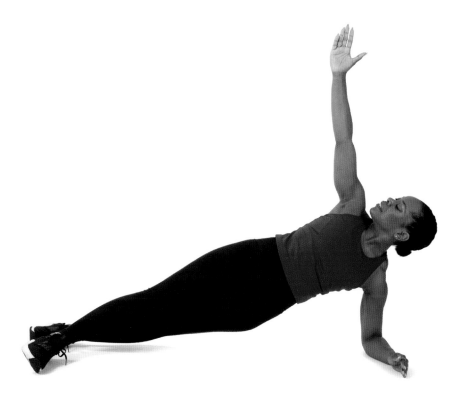

The first step in starting an exercise program is identifying your reasons for doing it. For example, why do you want to exercise your abs and glutes? What results do you want for your body? Is it to increase your workout intensity? Is it to improve your fitness and muscular endurance? Is it to develop an overall stronger core? Is it to develop the shape of your abs and glutes in some particular way? Different training modalities exist for each of those aspirations, so you need to know what you want in order to know how to get it.

Why Core Goals Are Personal

You are encouraged to have a specific goal for what you want to get out of your core training program before diving into a plan. Is it to add a specific focus to improve your workout routine for better overall health? Is it to alleviate low-back pain? Is it to improve your posture? Is it to improve your balance? Is it to get stronger? Is it to lose size? Is it to gain mass and muscle size?

As you start to develop a specific, measurable goal for yourself and your core training program, keep these important concepts in mind:

• *Be real, and keep it real with yourself.* Be realistic with your goal setting. Safely and healthily approach your fitness pace. While muscle fatigue and soreness may be immediately apparent, it takes weeks and sometimes months to experience noticeable changes to your physique. Another part of being realistic is not comparing yourself to others; doing so doesn't support your mental or physical health.

• *Know that spot reduction is a farce.* Targeting a specific area of the body does not mean you will burn fat in just that area. Instead, your body burns fat distributed throughout your body. Be grateful for the body you have. Although focused training can have benefits, such as muscle development as discussed in this book, training for overall health and functionality will always reign supreme.

• *Keep in mind that genetics plays a role in your body composition.* Genetics are a factor in body composition and body size, and therefore impact the general shape of the body. Everyone is made differently. Your physical makeup largely depends on your genes, environment, and behavioral patterns. The combination of genetics, diet, and behavioral environment (which includes exercise patterns) influences your fitness results. If round butts and slim waists don't run in your family but this is a look you want, you can use exercise to make gains in that direction.

• *Remember that abs are made in the kitchen.* As trite as it may sound, this statement has some truth to it. Proper nutrition combined with consistent exercise engagement will help uncover the washboard abs that you already have but may not be able to see. Certain foods and meal plans can boost metabolism, burn excess fat, and improve satiety after meal consumption. It is best to consult with a professional such as a registered dietician to set your unique and personal meal plan based on your goals. Every body is made differently, therefore each one responds to nutritional plans and exercise plans differently. Exercise is not a one-size-fits-all prescription; pay close attention to your own journey and goals, and seek advice specific to your anatomical needs and desires.

Setting personalized goals before pursuing any exercise plan is an efficient way to set yourself up for success because it saves you time, effort, and disappointment. Plenty of available exercise programs offer a generalized approach to fitness. However, keep in mind that bodies are not all the same and therefore they don't all respond equally. Even if two people were to follow the exact same plans, results would still vary.

Nutritional Rule to Remember

To support good health and proper body function, eat foods with a balance of high-quality fat, carbohydrate, and protein. Balancing a wide range of nutrients helps you to reduce risk of disease, maintain a healthy weight, and power your exercise journey.

Rather than follow a workout plan because you want to look like the actor or model who does it, a better goal is to find a program that helps you feel, perform, and look like a better version of you, for you, and based on your own standards and desires. When you first accept and appreciate the body you have, you can set achievable goals and enjoy real rewards.

Prepare yourself for the exercises and workouts in this book by first answering these important questions:

- What do I really want to accomplish?
- What are my goals, and why do I want to achieve them?
- Are those goals truly realistic and achievable for my body?

The following section is intended to help you clearly identify your goals.

Goal-Setting Basics

Motivation is a key factor in setting personal goals. The goals that you set should be of enough value and importance to you that you strive to achieve the desired outcome. Goal achievement requires commitment, focus, accountability, consistency, and priority. When you're setting goals, remember the acronym SMART:

- **S**pecific
- **M**easurable
- **A**ttainable
- **R**elevant
- **T**imely

Set a *specific* goal that is precise and well defined. It will help you develop a clear road map for where you intend to go or what you plan to achieve. For example, a goal might be, *I want to gain muscle mass.* Using this example, you can narrow down this baseline goal with the rest of the SMART method for goal setting.

Make sure the goal is *measurable*, perhaps numerically by target date, volume of repetitions (reps), weight gain or loss, or muscle mass gain or loss. This measure should be precise. For example, an ambiguous goal such as *Gain muscle mass* becomes *Increase muscle mass by 2 percent within 12 weeks*.

Set a goal that is *attainable*. In other words, keep it real. If it is impossible to achieve your goal, you will lose faith in the process and confidence in yourself. Gaining 2 percent muscle mass in 12 weeks may be a healthy and doable goal, whereas gaining 10 percent muscle mass in a shorter period of time is impractical and nearly impossible.

Set *relevant* goals that align with what you desire for yourself. A goal that has relevance is more practical and attainable, so pinpoint the why—the reason the goal is important to you. For example, the goal *I want to obtain a tighter core and stronger, larger glute muscles so that I feel more confident in my clothes next vacation, because I personally like that look* includes relevance. When you pinpoint the reason the goal is important to you, you will help make it more relevant and purposeful.

To set a *timely* goal, make sure you have a time frame for which you expect to achieve it. A deadline creates a sense of urgency and importance, and a finish line creates an opportunity for celebration. Having timely goals increases the likelihood that you will stick to them until you see them come to fruition.

Now, list the goals you want to reach (see the SMART Goal Setting form in figure 3.1). No matter the number of goals, remember to follow the SMART method for each goal. Plan to work on one goal first, then move on to the next one. You may also want to have short-term (less than 6 months) and long-term (more than 6 months) goals; be sure to plan the steps you need to take to meet them.

Now that you have answered important questions relevant to your goal setting (the *what* and the *why*), prepare to dive deeper into the *how* of approaching your goals.

Picking the best training options for your body is ideal for reaching achievable goals.

Factors responsible for the outcome of individual exercise training programs include the following:

- *Sex*: The biological difference between male and female sexes and the role it plays in exercise intensity
- *Age*: Choosing age-appropriate exercise, which means finding the appropriate exercise options based on age, cognitive development, and physical abilities that correlate with aging
- *Current fitness level*: Present-day fitness or physical abilities—not memories of athleticism of the past or possibilities of the future
- *Exercise history*: Past engagement in exercise and how that engagement relates to muscle memory and your own know-how with specific movement patterns

SMART Goal Setting

Goal 1:

_____

_____

_____

_____

Goal 2:

_____

_____

_____

_____

Goal 3:

_____

_____

_____

_____

Goal 4:

_____

_____

_____

_____

Goal 5:

_____

_____

_____

_____

FIGURE 3.1   Form for SMART goal setting.

From K. Williams, _Functional Core for Women_ (Champaign, IL: Human Kinetics, 2024).

- *Genetics*: How the body will adapt to a certain type of exercise, such as cardiorespiratory fitness, muscular strength, and explosive power
- *Rest and recovery periods*: Necessary components for the body to repair itself and experience beneficial results
- *Nutrition*: Fueling the body with food to affect fitness performance and bodily changes
- *Hydration*: Fueling the body with fluid to affect how the body performs, recovers, and sleeps
- *Other emotional, psychological, and physical stressors in life, work, and relationships*: Factors that affect whether you feel like exercising and how well you actually engage in exercise

Following are tips to increase workout intensity:

- Increase load by adding more resistance or weight to the exercise to make each rep more muscularly challenging. To increase load, you can use resistance bands, weighted exercise balls, or tubing with greater resistance. You can also use heavier dumbbells or barbells. Increasing load can also aid in building *muscular strength* (the amount of force you can exert for a short period).
- Decrease rest time between exercise sets, which will require your body to adapt more quickly to the exercise demand.
- Increase exercise volume by adding more sets or reps for the exercise. This increase will target the already fatigued muscles with an extra push—as long as you can perform the added reps safely and with optimal form. It can also improve *muscular endurance* (the ability of a muscle to withstand exercise time under tension, such as added resistance or body weight, for a period of time).
- Train both unilaterally and bilaterally, which are equally effective ways to intensify any exercise and challenge strength and power. A *unilateral* exercise movement is when each side or limb of your body works independently of the other, such as a single-leg squat or single-leg hip bridge. A *bilateral* exercise movement is when both limbs work in unison to perform a given exercise, such as a traditional squat with both feet on the ground. Typically, a unilateral exercise seems more challenging because it requires more of a balance challenge to your core stability. However, a bilateral exercise can be just as challenging when you focus on performing the exercise optimally, change the tempo, or add resistance.

Following are tips to increase strength and add lean muscle development:

- Increase the workload for an exercise. You can increase the number of sets or reps performed to put more demand on the muscles.

Adding resistance is another way to increase workload. The heavier or more taxing the resistance, the fewer safe and effective reps your body will be able to perform of a given exercise set before fatigue or failure.

- Increase time under tension, which extends the amount of time it takes to perform a given exercise set. (The term *time under tension* refers to the amount of time that a muscle is under stress or tension.) You can slow the movement and spend more time during the more challenging phase of the given exercise.

- Change up the tempo by lengthening or shortening the amount of time during the concentric (when the muscle contracts) or eccentric (when the muscle lengthens) phase of the exercise or both. For example, you might try squatting down slowly and coming up quickly, or vice versa; or slowly go down and slowly come up. You can mix up your tempos.

- Add an isometric hold to an exercise set. During an isometric hold, the targeted muscle(s) do not change length and the nearest joint does not move. For example, try holding a lunge for a few seconds at the bottom of the movement.

Following are tips to improve muscular endurance:

- Increase the number of reps performed with optimal form and alignment until muscular fatigue. You could also add an additional rep to each set of a given exercise.

- Lower the amount of weight or resistance in order to perform more reps.

- Increase the duration that you are active in an exercise; for example, hold a plank for an additional number of seconds each time you perform the plank.

Following are tips to encourage hypertrophy (increasing muscle mass or size):

- For muscular gains, you need significant tension and metabolic stress on the muscles being targeted. One way to accomplish this goal is to add significantly heavier resistance to the exercise—as long as you can perform the exercise safely.

- Lift strong and heavy weight until muscular fatigue. It is necessary to create muscle fiber tears and repairs and exhaust adenosine triphosphate (ATP, an energy component that helps the muscle contract) to increase muscle size. In other words, you have to work against heavy resistance to the point that you cannot properly perform another rep under that amount of tension.

- Employ progressive overload (gradually increase intensity or difficulty) to develop muscle mass. This can be done by increasing resistance, decreasing rest periods, adding repetitions or weights, or changing exercise tempo. Create exercise tempo changes by lengthening the concentric phase and shortening the eccentric phase. For example, when performing a hip bridge, take two to four seconds to lift up (concentric phase; glute muscles are shortening/contracting) and take one to three seconds to lower down (eccentric phase; glutes are lengthening), or vice versa.

- Recovery is essential for muscle growth and development, so allow yourself rest days (muscle repairing days) between days of heavy resistance training. For example, lift heavy two or three days a week; either rest or focus on other muscle groups on the days between.

Goal setting adds purpose, value, functionality, and a road map to success. To make progress and eventually get to where you want to go on your core exercise journey, first set personal goals using the SMART method and then create a clear plan to accomplish them. Then comes the workout. The following chapter guides you in developing your exercise program.

CHAPTER 4

Developing Your Core Program

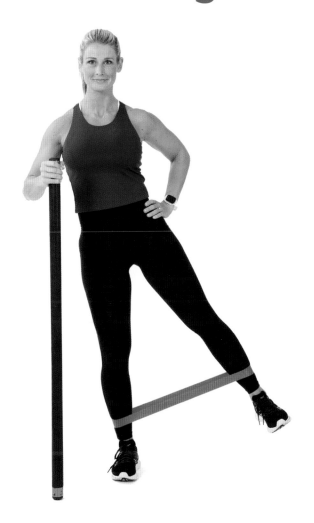

When developing your personal exercise program, the scientific principles of training can effectively guide you to improve your exercise performance and maximize your target results.

An Ode to Core

Oh, my dear core, the central part of me,
A system of muscles, some too deep to see.
To stabilize and support my body in motion,
To train and exercise, I give you my devotion.
Muscles that twist and turn,
Chisel and burn,
Strengthen and lengthen,
And, oh yeah extension.
Responsible for so much movement,
Functional, big, and sometimes small.
Many tools and tips for self-improvement,
This is my tribute to you, at the core of it all.

Think of these principles as your tools for success that help you elevate your exercise experience. As you prepare for internal and external, feel-good and look-good results, it's worth the effort to first understand these tools.

Core Training Tools

This book explores many exercise options that focus on your abs and glutes. It also introduces various pieces of exercise equipment and accessories that you can use for the recommended exercises. These pieces can make a movement more or less challenging for you, so listen to your body when deciding what to use. For effective results and injury prevention, your form, alignment, and movement technique should be solid before adding equipment and toys to your exercise training. Tools for core training include the following:

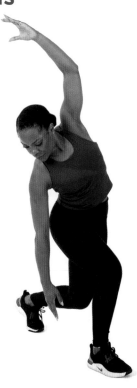

- **Body weight**
  - Nature's most portable and accessible exercise tool, body weight is commonly used in all exercises.
  - You can do all the exercises in this book solely with body weight; no additional equipment is necessary.

- **Resistance bands**
  - Made of latex or synthetic rubber and coming in various resistance levels, these elastic bands can be integrated into various exercises for added resistance and strength challenges.
  - They are optional for use in glute-focused exercises such as lateral squats and hip bridges with abduction.

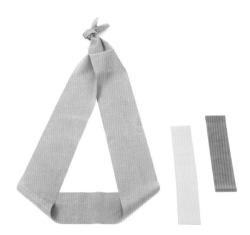

- **Resistance tubing**
  - A versatile strength-challenging tool with handles, tubing is commonly used to pull and press against. It is made for different levels of added tension in movement.
  - It is optional for use in glute-focused exercises such as quadruped leg extensions.

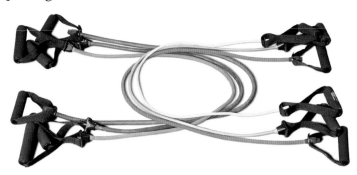

- **Weighted fitness bar**
  - This weighted, one-piece fitness tool is commonly used for versatile weightlifting exercises.
  - It is optional for use in providing stability (held vertically and anchored on the floor for balance support).

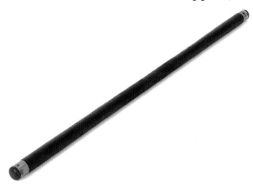

- **Exercise gliders or sliders**
  - A disc-shaped exercise tool designed to be placed under the hands or feet, gliders provide a smooth sliding surface for an added layer of challenge to body-weight exercises. These can also be substituted with paper plates. Use them to find additional length and strength in the active phase of various exercises.
  - They are optional for use in glute-focused exercises such as supine leg extensions and ab-focused exercises such as moving planks.

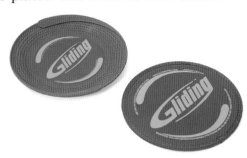

- **Dome-like balance trainer**
  - This fitness accessory is great for an added challenge to balance, strength, and flexibility. You can use it with the dome-side up or dome-side down with caution.
  - It is optional for use in glute-focused exercises such as squats and lunges and ab-focused exercises such as planks and bicycle.

- **Barbell**
  - Used in weight training, this equipment consists of a long bar, usually with weight plates on either end of the bar. It is commonly used for added resistance and additional muscular challenge and building.
  - It is optional for use in body-weight exercises such as squats, lunges, and hip bridges.

- **Dumbbells and kettlebells**
  - This portable free-weight equipment is used for weight and resistance training. It is effective for added muscular challenge and building.

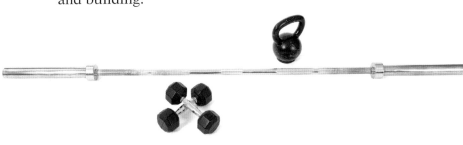

- Dumbbells and kettlebells are optional for use in ab-focused exercises such as Russian twist and glute-focused exercises such as donkey kick.
- **Medicine ball**
    - Also known as med ball, exercise ball, fitness ball, or weighted ball, a medicine ball is a ball filled with sand or other material for added weight. It is used for strength training and to improve neuromuscular coordination.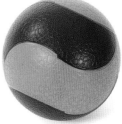
    - It is optional for use in ab-focused exercises such as sit-ups.

Six Principles of Training

The following training principles help with exercise adaptations, progressions, and improvements in your fitness training and performance: specificity, individuality, progressive overload, variation, diminishing return, and reversibility. They are defined and discussed next.

1. *Specificity*: Your exercise training program should be specific to the goals you hope to achieve. For example, if the goal is to build muscle mass, your program should include lifting weights instead of only going for long-distance runs. This principle does not apply to a goal of general fitness.

2. *Individuality*: Your fitness journey is unlike anyone else's. Having a training partner is great, especially for accountability and socialization, but it does not mean you both will perform the same and have the same results. Your exercise program should be specific to your needs, goals, and abilities. Also, your body and fitness level will not be the same every day. Some days are harder than others. On some days, you feel stronger than on other days. Take heed and be patient with yourself.

3. *Progressive overload*: Your body will respond to exercise persistence and consistency by way of getting stronger and having more endurance. Gradually and safely, in small increments over time, increasing frequency, intensity, time, and type of exercise programming (known as the FITT principle) is ideal for continuously making gains and for fitness longevity.

4. *Variation*: Adding variety to your training program can have positive results and will keep you from getting bored. If you find yourself hitting a plateau or becoming unmotivated after doing the same workout time after time, mix it up. Try different equipment, use different ranges and planes of motion, and add circuit or high-intensity interval training (HIIT) exercise programs.

5. *Diminishing return*: This principle means you hit a workout plateau or no longer receive the same growth and progress from a workout you have been doing. Working to remain mentally and physically stimulated lessens the likelihood of experiencing diminishing return. Push through the plateau by varying your exercise program, avoiding overtraining, and getting sufficient rest and recovery. Your rest days are important. Avoid overtraining, which has an adverse effect on your fitness journey. You build muscle and strength while recovering from the work you did during your workout. The best body adaptation to exercise comes with adequate rest.

6. *Reversibility*: When you stop exercising, fitness gains can reverse course and turn into losses. Think of the phrase *Use it or lose it*. Drastically dropping off from your exercise frequency or not exercising for weeks at a time will result in you losing all the fitness gains you made when you were working out consistently. Remember that consistency is key. Stick to your routine, and sustainable results will come.

As you prepare to develop a program that is specific to your goals, keep in mind the FITT principle—frequency, intensity, time, and type of exercise—as follows:

- Decide the *frequency* (how often you will train). Perhaps you want to strive for two or three days a week of vigorous or intense exercise. Maybe your fitness level and schedule are more suited for three to five days of moderate exercise at minimum.

- Choose your *intensity* (how hard you want to train). Consider the workload, the amount of resistance, the number of sets and reps, the amount of time under tension (TUT), and how taxing the exercise time will be on your body. Moderate to vigorous intensity is recommended for most adults.

- Decide on how much *time* you will dedicate to each workout session. An ideal goal for the average adult exerciser is 30 to 60 minutes each day.

- Decide what *type* of exercise training program you will commit to for a given time. For general and well-balanced fitness goals, it is recommended that most adults engage in a combination of cardiorespiratory, strength, and flexibility training throughout each week.

Exercise Selection

It is important to learn to perform exercises optimally and make sure you are selecting the appropriate exercises for your body, fitness level, and goals. Consider the purpose and the goals of each exercise before doing them, and note how or what you should feel when performing each exercise. This awareness will help you to train safely, more effectively, and with intention.

Focus on optimal form. There is no such thing as perfect form; perfection is unattainable. Another idea to challenge is so-called correct form. No one correct form exists because each body is different. However, using *optimal* form is a best practice that works for your body type and is unique to your motor learning. Performing any exercise should not result in injury, so be cautious and stay aware of your personal form.

Exercise variation, weight selection, and the use of accessories could facilitate progression or regression of an exercise move. Sometimes the traditional version of an exercise is not right for you. You are encouraged to address weakness and imbalances to improve your movement pattern, but sometimes performing a variation of an exercise is the key for you to feel accomplished and reach your ideal success.

An exercise program does not have to be complicated to be effective, and choosing too many exercises can be inefficient for progress. It is all about quality over quantity. Never sacrifice optimal form in any given exercise. Once optimal form starts to weaken, you should end the exercise. Consider choosing a variety of exercises and ordering them in a sensible way that makes up your unique program. Here are some suggestions for selecting and organizing your exercise program:

1. *Do exercises for so-called problem muscles (the more troubling muscles of your focused training or specific exercises that you least desire to do) first*. It is best to perform these exercises at the beginning of the exercise program to prevent skipping them at the end of the workout and avoid fatigue-related injuries. Get them done while you have the greatest amount of effort, energy, attention, and focus available.

2. *Multijoint exercises should come before single-joint or isolation exercises*. Essentially, the squat, lunge, and leg press, which incorporate hips, knees, and ankles, should come before an isolated move such as the hamstring curl, leg extension, or lateral leg raise. Multijoint exercises help maximize strength in larger muscle groups; burn more calories; and improve balance, coordination, flexibility, and preparation for isolation exercises. Isolation exercises are where definition and sculpting of a specific muscle happens.

3. *Target larger muscle groups before smaller muscle groups*. Exercises that target larger muscles groups (e.g., lats, glutes, quads) should come before those targeting smaller or accessory muscles (e.g., biceps, obliques, rectus abdominis) because larger muscle groups are responsible for the major movements and strength that help activate smaller muscle groups. Essentially, you will work the glutes before moving your focus to the abs because more often than not, the abs are activated and working as stabilizers in all other exercises being performed anyway.

4. *Exercises with added weight such as dumbbells and barbells (also called free weights) should come before exercises with sectorized resistance machines and resistance bands.* This order promotes safety in an exercise program because exercises performed with free weights call for more energy expenditure and motor control than exercises performed on machines that assist with movement control, especially when the muscles are starting to fatigue toward the end of the workout.

5. *Change the angles of exercises for a single target muscle group performed in succession.* This approach provides more complete development of the muscle group. For example, in ab- and glute-focused exercises, try these variations: change your limb placement from wide or narrow to split; or change your body placement from flat, incline, or decline to supine, prone, or side lying. The changes will create variety, and they will challenge and develop the muscles from all angles.

The general goal of glute training, depending on intensity, is two to four times a week with three to six different exercises and angles. The general goal for abdominal muscle development is a minimum of four different exercises in different angles two or three times a week. However, abs and glutes can easily be incorporated into other exercise programming or a full-body workout. Essentially, like any other muscle, you can train two or three times a week while staying mindful of the importance of rest and recovery.

A developed program is a plan for success. Affording yourself the opportunity to front-load your training journey with a planning stage will result in a clear road map for success and for achieving your exercise and fitness goals.

PART III

EXERCISES

CHAPTER 5

Standing Core Exercises

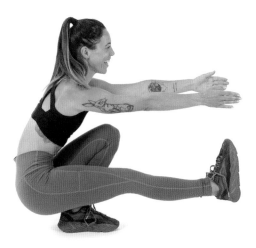

The number of hours you spend sitting each day may be alarming. Sitting for prolonged periods has a negative effect on gluteal muscle activation and body posture. Standing recruits and strengthens muscles of the abs, back, glutes, and legs, and it burns more calories than sitting. Why not add intentional exercises performed while standing to double up on the benefits?

Standing core exercises come in many forms and styles, so you can use them to mix up your regular training routine. A perk of standing core exercises is that you burn more calories in less time because you engage more muscles at once. Also, standing core exercises can be functional; they challenge your balance and stability while improving your posture. Finally, if you experience pain in the neck or hip flexors when doing core exercises on the floor, standing core exercises will be a welcomed alternative for you.

Keep in mind that training to make your glutes and abs pop takes time and commitment to your exercise program and diet; results will not happen overnight. Proper nutrition and strategic exercise goals will help to strengthen and define your core muscles and reduce the layer of body fat that covers them. Also remember that for safety, it is best to do all core exercises in a controlled and efficient manner that will not make you susceptible to injury.

The following standing core exercises will help improve your focus, functional strength, balance, posture, and physique.

SQUAT

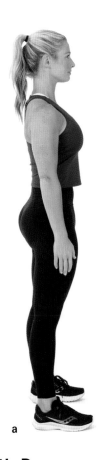

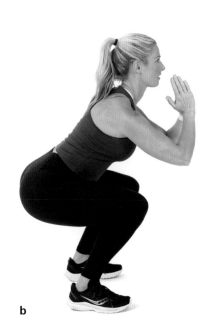

a   b

How It's Done

1. Stand with the feet a little wider than hip width and the toes and knees facing forward.
2. Keeping the belly muscles strong, push the hips back, bend the knees and ankles, and press the knees slightly open as you lower as if to sit.
3. Sit into a squat position while keeping the heels and toes on the ground, chest up, and shoulders back.
4. Work to bring the thighs parallel to the ground; knees are bent at a 90-degree angle.
5. Pressing the heels into the ground, straighten the legs to return to a standing position.
6. Repeat for repetitions.

Regressions and Progressions

1. Decrease range of motion by staying above parallel with the thighs.
2. Increase range of motion by sitting lower in the squat.
3. Challenge core stability and balance by performing your squats on an unstable surface such as a dome-like balance trainer or other balance training equipment.

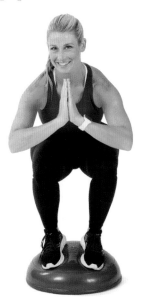

Safety Cues

1. Remember to actively engage the abs and keep the chest lifted and proud. This exercise should not cause pain in your lower back; if you experience pain, you may have lowered too far and exceeded your current range of motion.
2. Keep the heels connected with the floor at all times.
3. Keep the knees behind the toes.

Variations

1. To further challenge, add weight on the shoulder, at chest height, or at the sides of the body.
2. Perform squats with bands around the thighs, and actively push the knees open to help improve your squat mechanics and strengthen the abductors (the muscles that rotate the legs to the side and away from the midline of the body).

SQUAT TAPBACK

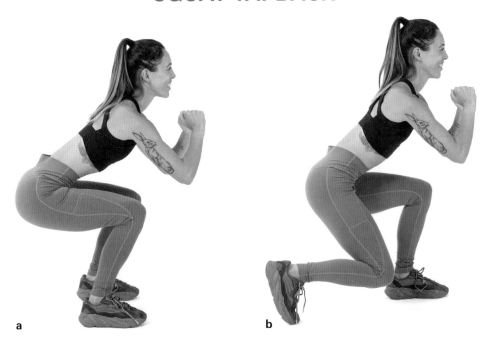

a   b

How It's Done

1. In a squat position, tap one foot back—about 1 to 2 feet (30-60 cm) behind you.
2. Return the foot to the original starting position, then switch to the other side.
3. Remain low in the squat position the entire time as you alternate from tapping one foot back to the other.

Regressions and Progressions

1. Decrease range of motion by keeping the thighs above parallel and taking shorter steps back.
2. Increase range of motion by lowering farther in your squat and tapping farther back.

Safety Cues

1. Avoid bouncing at the knees. Bouncing could add unnecessary strain and injury to the joints.
2. Actively keep the core muscles engaged and strong.
3. As you tap back, gently tap the big toe back rather than planting the entire foot down.

Variations

1. Add resistance bands either above the knees or just above the ankles for added resistance challenge.
2. Do a squat back-leg lift: Rather than tap the toes back, straighten and lift the back leg 1 to 2 feet (30-60 cm) from the floor, engaging the glutes as you lift for additional challenge.
3. Perform this exercise with a figure-8 tubing under your feet for additional challenge and resistance.

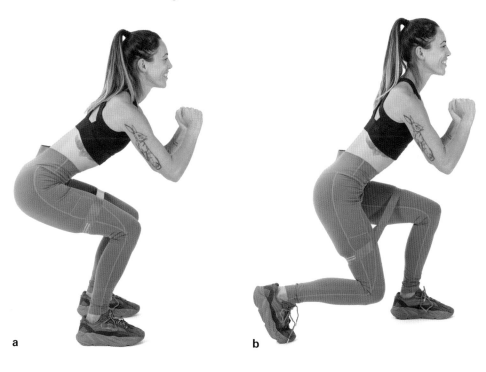

a
b

GLUTES

LUNGE

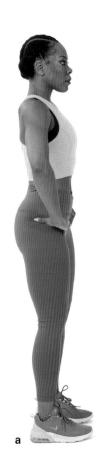

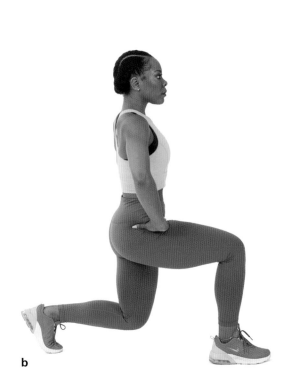

a   b

How It's Done

1. Start by standing up tall with the hands at the hips.
2. Take a big step forward with one foot.
3. Bend the knees and ankles, lowering the body until the knees and ankles each flex at a 90-degree angle. Keep the back heel lifted from the floor.
4. Lift the front lunging leg, and step it back to return to the starting position.
5. Repeat for repetitions or switch sides.

Regressions and Progressions

1. Shorten your range of motion by not going down as low or by staying above a 90-degree angle at the knees.
2. Find greater range of motion by actively working to get lower in the lunge position.

Safety Cues

1. Be sure to step far enough forward so that you are able to bend the front knee without the knee passing the toes.
2. Keep the toes and knees on both sides aligned and forward in the lunging position.
3. Keep the shoulders back and chest up so that you are not bowing the torso forward as you lunge.

Variations

1. Do a reverse lunge to knee to engage the abs and other core muscles on the concentric working phase.
2. Do a forward lunge to knee to encourage longer stepping and active hip flexors.
3. Do a reverse lunge to forward lunge for added agility and coordination work.
4. Lunge onto or off of a piece of equipment that creates instability for balance challenge.
5. Use resistance bands for added muscular challenge.

DEADLIFT

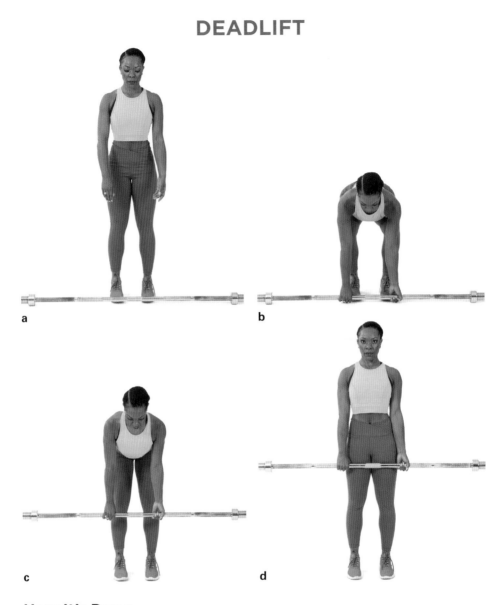

a

b

c

d

How It's Done

1. Stand behind a barbell with the mid foot under the bar, feet about hip-width apart.

2. Bend the knees and hinge at the hips so that you are able to grab the bar with straight arms using an overhand, underhand, or split grip; keep the shoulders and hips aligned at a straight angle (not rounding in the back).

3. With a firm grip on the bar and keeping the shoulders back and down, activate all core muscles. Press both entire feet into the ground, and lift the torso and straighten the back while pulling the weight as you rise up to a standing position.

4. Keep the same form as you hinge at the hips, bend the knees slightly, push the butt way back, and lower the barbell to shin height with the back nearly parallel to the ground.

5. Repeat for repetitions.

Regressions and Progressions

1. For a regression, decrease your range of motion by not lowering the bar as far down.

2. With optimal form, find greater depth by lowering the barbell to the ankles or mid foot or to the ground.

Safety Cues

1. Squaring the hips and shoulders and engaging the abs are key for protecting the back while performing a deadlift.

2. Keep the hips back on the eccentric phase of the exercise.

3. Keep the knees slightly bent and arms straight.

4. Flex the muscles of the back and armpits when pulling the weight from the dead position.

Variations

1. Perform the kickstand deadlift to create instability in the body and help train your balance more by staggering your stance.

2. The single-leg deadlift is a progression from the kickstand deadlift; balancing on one leg requires even more control and core stability.

3. Perform the offset-load deadlift with a dumbbell in one hand to create instability in the body and challenge your stabilizing muscles more.

4. Perform other deadlift variations with kettlebells, dumbbells, or elastic bands for challenging resistance and equipment variations.

5. Do a deadlift using gliders to recruit muscular adaptation to movement and instability.

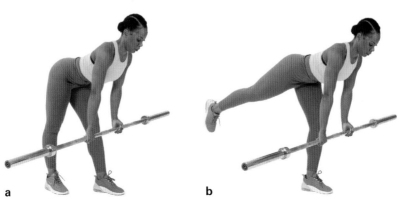

a   b

SUMO DEADLIFT

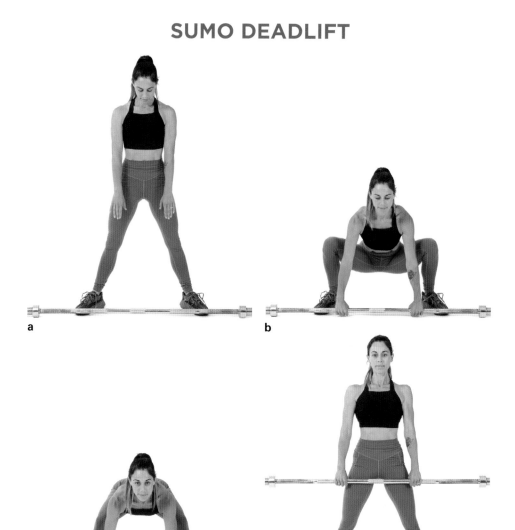

a

b

c

d

How It's Done

1. Approach the barbell close enough so that you do not reach out or forward for the bar. You should be able to reach straight down and touch the bar.

2. Stand with the feet wider than shoulder-width apart, toes and knees turned out, lifting through the arches of the feet, and knees slightly bent. Foot placement is personal, so find an angle that feels right for your hips, knees, and ankles.

3. Hinging at the hips, bend the knees to lower your body. The torso should be almost parallel to the floor; pushing the butt far back, keep the shoulders and hips square without rounding the back (flat-back position). Take hold of the barbell overhand, underhand, or with a split grip.

4. Keeping the core tight, look slightly forward and up, then push through the heels to return to standing upright. Keep the barbell directly under the body as you pull.

5. To lower the barbell back to the floor, bend the knees with the butt pushed back, the torso in a neutral spinal position, and the arms fully extended.

6. Repeat for repetitions.

Regressions and Progressions

1. Decrease the amount of weight on the barbell.

2. Add heavier weights to the barbell.

Safety Cues

1. The sumo position allows you to get lower to the ground due to the wide positioning of the legs and feet, which helps to lessen the urge to round the back.

2. Keep the feet far apart and the knees aligned with the second or third toe on each foot. The knees should not bow inward.

3. Do not round the back.

4. Make sure shoes are tied tightly so that the feet are not sliding around in your shoes and the heels remain on the floor during the exercise.

Variations

1. Create more turnout (a greater degree of external rotation at the hip joint), with the toes and knees open outward more, to increase work for the inner thighs.

2. Hold a dumbbell or kettlebell hanging at the dead position in the center of the legs for more muscular challenge.

3. Wear a tight resistance band at thigh height to build strength in the deep rotators and length in the inner thighs for improving turnout.

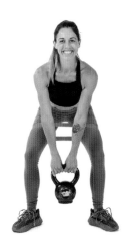

SUMO SQUAT

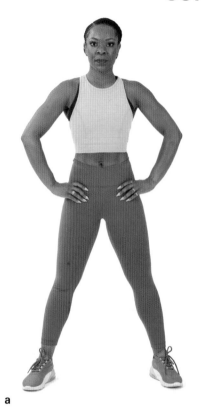
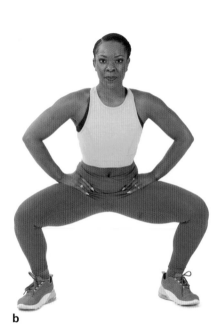

a   b

How It's Done

1. Stand with the feet wider than shoulder-width apart and the hips externally rotated so that the toes and knees are diagonally turned out at about a 45-degree angle, and lift through the arches of the feet. The chest is lifted and proud, the shoulders are back, and the hips are aligned under shoulders.

2. Bend the knees, pushing the knees out to align with the second or third toe on each foot; the knees do not pass the toes. At the bottom of the squat, you should be able to see the insides of your feet.

3. The chest and spine should remain upright as you lower your body down, stopping once the thighs reach a position that is parallel to the floor. The heels remain connected with the floor. If the heels lift, perhaps you have lowered too far for your range of motion.

4. Keeping the abs engaged, the spine long and tall, and the weight in the heels as you engage the glutes and inner thighs, return to standing.

5. Repeat for repetitions.

Regressions and Progressions

1. Decrease range of motion on the depth of the squat and on the foot placement and turnout.
2. To intensify the muscular challenge, hold weights at the chest, down in front of the body, or on the shoulders.

Safety Cues

1. The sumo squat position does not require you to actively push the hips back as in a parallel-stance squat. Be mindful that you do not hinge at the hips or bow forward as you would in a sumo deadlift; sumo squat and sumo deadlift are not the same exercise.
2. Keep the feet far apart; the knees align with the second or third toe on each foot and should not bow in. Pull the knees back.
3. Do not round the back, but keep the chest lifted and proud. Keep the shoulders stacked over the hips, and stand relatively upright for the entire time.

Variations

1. Increase turnout; the greater your turnout, the more emphasis you place on the inner thighs.
2. Use resistance bands for additional abduction conditioning.
3. Do the sumo squat on an unstable, lifted surface such as a step or dome-like balance trainer to create imbalance and challenge stability.

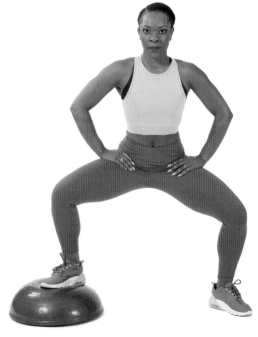

LATERAL LUNGE

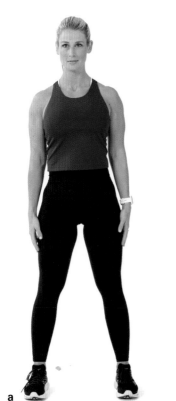
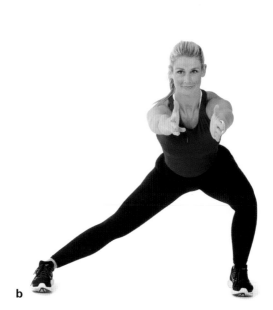

a   b

How It's Done

1. Stand tall with the feet parallel, shoulders stacked over hips, hips stacked over heels, and abs engaged.

2. Take a wide step to the side. Land with the entire foot on the ground, ensuring the torso is as upright as possible. Bend the knee of the leading leg toward a 90-degree angle while keeping the trailing leg extended.

3. Push off the heel and ball of the foot, actively engage the adductors (muscles of the hip that bring the thighs toward the midline of the body) to lift back up, and return to the starting position.

4. Repeat for repetitions or switch sides.

Regressions and Progressions

1. Shorten the step out to the side as a regression.
2. Add weight or increase the width of the step and the depth of the lunge to add challenge.

Safety Cues

1. The toes and knees on both sides should remain aligned and forward in the lunging position. A slight turnout is acceptable.
2. Keep the shoulders back, chest lifted, and abs engaged so that you are not bowing as you lunge.

Variations

1. Add weight for more muscular challenge, such as dumbbells.
2. Use a glider; place the center of the active foot on the center of the glider for more stability and agility challenge.

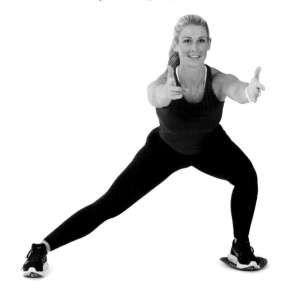

GLUTES

PISTOL SQUAT

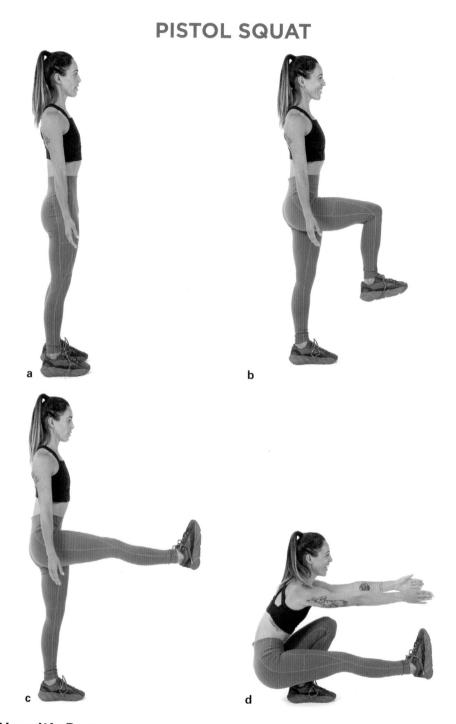

How It's Done

1. Stand tall with the feet parallel, toes pointed forward, shoulders stacked over hips, hips stacked over heels, and abs braced.
2. Lift one foot so that you are standing on one leg. Fully extend it in front of you so that the quad and ankle are flexed.

3. Stand strong and stable, and grip the floor with the entire foot of the standing leg.

4. Hinge at the hips, bend the standing knee, and sit the hips back while leaning the torso slightly forward to counterbalance the squat and aid in balance.

5. Lower as far down and as confidently as possible, keeping the core engaged and the ankle stabilized; one leg and both arms are extended in front of the torso.

6. Keeping your balance, push the standing foot into the ground and place the extended leg next to the standing leg as you return to standing upright.

7. Repeat for repetitions or switch sides.

Regressions and Progressions

1. For a regression, sit back on a stabilized, high surface, like a plyometrics box, or hold on to a weighted fitness bar or barbell to aid in balance and provide other contact points to ground through when returning to standing.

2. For a progression, increase the depth of your squat, or touch the fingers to the extended toes.

3. For an additional progression, add load, or increase time under tension (TUT).

Safety Cues

Move slowly, engage the core, and keep the entire foot planted during this unilateral strengthening exercise to help keep body control and joint stability.

Variations

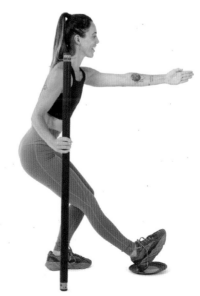

1. Sit back on a stabilized surface to deactivate muscles of the lower half, then reactivate to return to standing for more muscular challenge and to challenge stability and balance more.

2. Do a single-leg drop squat: Perform a single-leg squat while standing on an elevated surface or step with the inactive leg off the step for more stability challenge.

3. Use a glider or slider on the extended leg and a weighted fitness bar or barbell for support in the pistol squat.

GLUTES

STANDING LEG RAISE

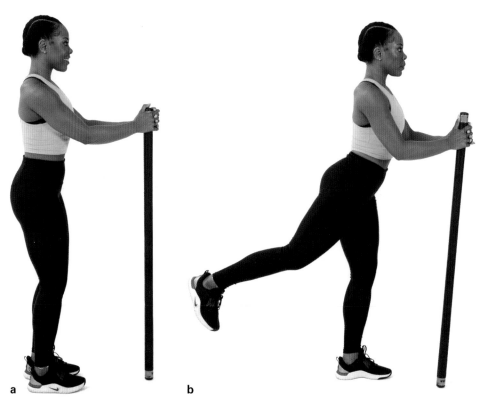

a   b

How It's Done

1. Stand tall with the shoulders back, chest up, and abs engaged, and softly bend the knees for a stable base. Firmly grip a weighted fitness bar or barbell for added stabilization.

2. Leading with the heel, lift one leg off the floor behind you as high as you can without bending that knee or arching the low back. Keep the torso upright.

3. With control, lower the leg to the starting position.

4. Repeat for repetitions or switch sides.

Regressions and Progressions

1. For a regression, stand more upright, and do not lift the leg as high.

2. For a progression, add an anchor point of resistance, and lean farther forward to protect the back while working against gravity and the added resistance.

Safety Cues

Keep the abs and stabilizing leg engaged to avoid a swayback posture when performing the move.

Variations

1. This exercise can be performed standing upright, kneeling on all fours, or lying in a prone position.
2. Add a resistance band; anchor the resistance band around the bar and the ankle of the moving leg for more resistance challenge.

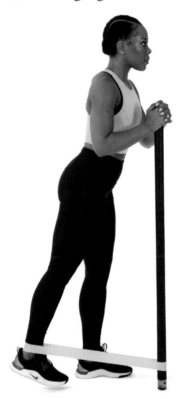

GLUTES

LATERAL LEG EXTENSION

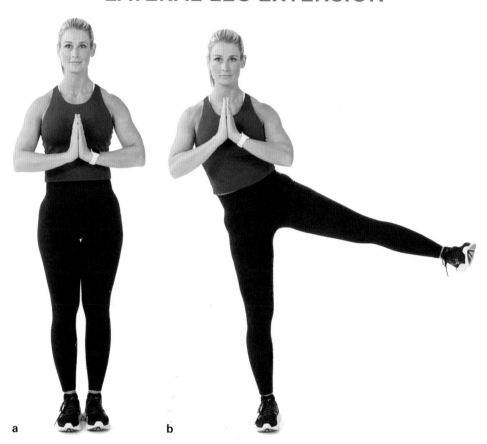

a   b

How It's Done

1. Stand tall with the shoulders back, chest up, and abs braced, arms placed at the sides or hands on hips or in prayer, and softly bend the knees for a stable base. Toes and knees are facing forward.

2. Shift your weight to one foot (standing leg). Flexing the other foot (lifting foot) and leading with the blade of that foot, lift the leg to the side as high as you can without bending the knee or leaning the torso to the side. Keep the torso upright.

3. With control, lower the leg, returning the foot to the starting position.

4. Repeat for repetitions or switch sides.

Regressions and Progressions

1. Hold on to a stable surface to help support balance for a regression.

2. For a progression, add a resistance band at the lower leg region to make the exercise more challenging.

Safety Cues

1. You do not have to lift your leg high for this move to be effective.
2. Keep your torso upright and legs long the entire time while performing this exercise.

Variations

1. This exercise can be performed standing upright, kneeling on all fours, or side lying on the floor if balance is a challenge.
2. Add a resistance band and a weighted fitness bar or barbell; loop the resistance band just above both ankles for added resistance while firmly gripping the bar for added balance support.

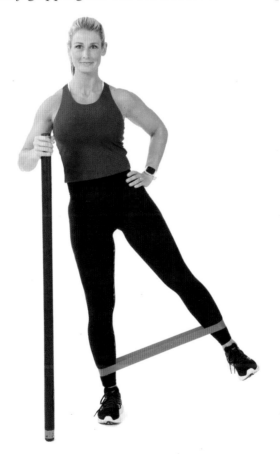

FORWARD FLEXION TO KNEE

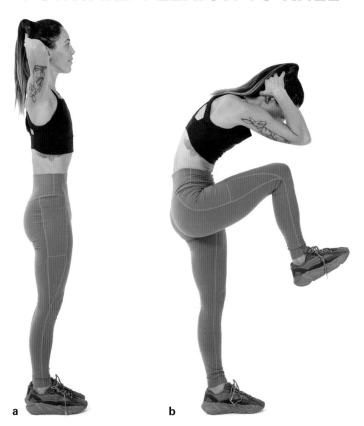

a   b

How It's Done

1. Stand tall with the shoulders back, chest up, and abs braced, and softly bend the knees for a stable base. Toes and knees are facing forward.

2. Place the hands behind the head with the fingers spread wide, thumbs at the nape of neck, and elbows wide.

3. Exhale as you crunch or flex forward, lifting one knee up toward the chest.

4. Inhale as you lower the leg, returning the foot to the starting position, standing upright with the chest lifted and proud.

5. Repeat for repetitions or switch sides.

Regressions and Progressions

1. Remain more upright and lessen the lift of the knee for a regression.
2. For a progression, lift the knee higher and round the torso, crunching or flexing more forward.

Safety Cues

1. Avoid pulling or tugging on the back of the head or neck.
2. Keep a bend in the stabilizing leg to help keep a solid base and balance.

Variations

1. Hold on to a stable surface for balance support.
2. Use a resistance band or tubing under both feet to create greater abdominal challenge as one leg raises.

ABS

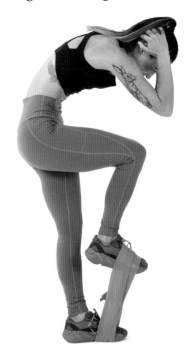

ABS

LATERAL FLEXION TO KNEE

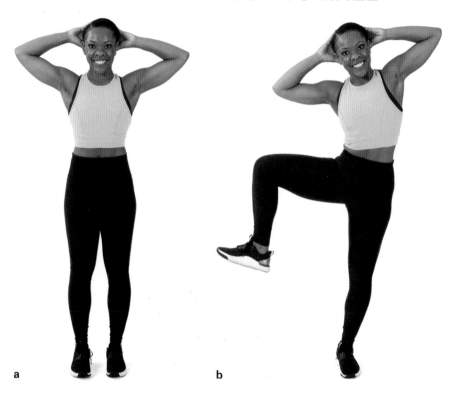

a   b

How It's Done

1. Stand tall with the shoulders back, chest up, and abs braced, and softly bend the knees for a stable base.
2. Place the hands behind the head, with the fingers spread wide, thumbs at the nape of the neck, and the elbows wide.
3. Exhale as you crunch, laterally flexing to the side, lifting one knee toward the same-side elbow. The foot and knee are turned out on the moving leg.
4. Inhale as you lower the leg, returning the foot to the starting position, standing upright with the chest lifted and proud.
5. Repeat for repetitions or switch sides.

Regressions and Progressions

1. Decrease the range of motion.
2. Increase the range of motion.

Safety Cues

1. Remember to stand tall the entire time, and avoid folding the torso forward during this exercise.
2. Keep the knees slightly bent to help with balance and control.

Variations

1. Hold on to a stable surface for balance support.
2. Use a resistance band or tubing under both feet to create more abdominal challenge as one leg raises.

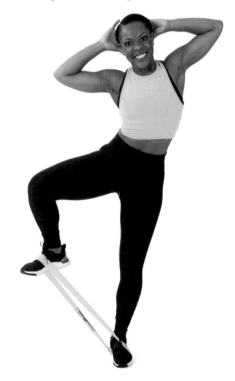

ABS

SUMO CROSSBODY REACH

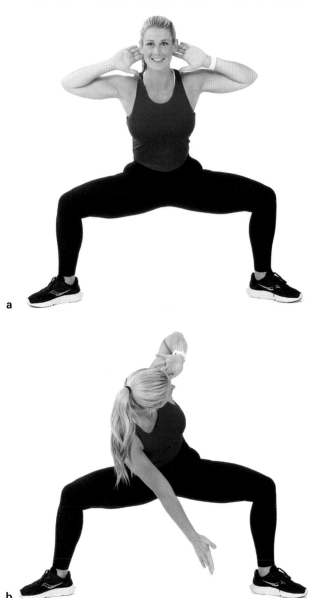

a

b

How It's Done

1. In a sumo squat position with the feet in a wide stance (wider than shoulder-width apart), turn out the toes and knees diagonally at about a 45-degree angle. With the chest lifted and proud, the shoulders back, and the hips aligned under the shoulders, lift through the arches of the feet, bending the knees toward a 90-degree angle.

2. Place both hands behind the head with the fingers spread wide, thumbs at the nape of the neck, and the elbows wide.

3. Rotating the torso, extend one arm across the midline of the body, reaching for the opposite ankle.

4. Keeping the abs engaged, lift the torso to return to the starting position.

5. Repeat for repetitions or switch sides.

Regressions and Progressions

1. Decrease the range of motion.
2. Increase the range of motion.

Safety Cues

Keep the shoulders back, chest lifted and proud, and knees back and aligned with the ankles the entire time.

Variations

1. Slow down the exercise to help keep body alignment and to prevent dizziness.
2. Use wrist weights for additional abdominal and shoulder muscle challenge.

ABS

ABS

CROSSBODY KNEE DRIVE

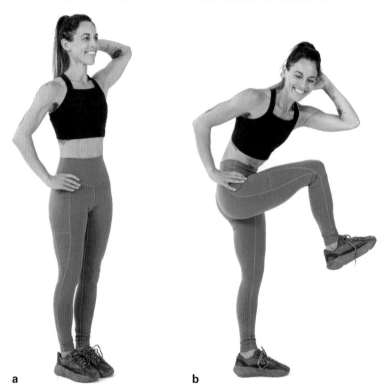

a   b

How It's Done

1. Stand tall with the shoulders back, chest lifted up, and abs braced, and softly bend the knees for a stable base. Toes and knees are facing forward.

2. Place one hand on the hip and the other behind the head with the fingers spread wide, thumb at the nape of neck, and elbow wide.

3. Exhale as you lift the knee opposite the hand that is behind the head, and twist the torso in the direction of the lifted knee, reaching the opposite knee and elbow across the midline toward each other.

4. Inhale as you lower the leg, returning the foot to the starting position, standing upright with the chest lifted and proud.

5. Repeat for repetitions or switch sides.

Regressions and Progressions

1. For a regression, shorten the range of motion, and slow the tempo.
2. For a progression, lift the knee higher while standing tall to recruit more abdominal muscles.

Safety Cues

1. Slow down the exercise tempo to maintain balance, alignment, and muscular control.
2. Remember to stand tall the entire time, and avoid folding the torso forward during this exercise.
3. When standing, keep the knees slightly bent to help with balance and control.

Variations

1. Hold on to a stable surface for balance support.
2. Slow down the exercise to help keep body alignment and to prevent dizziness.
3. Use a resistance band or tubing under the feet for added resistance challenge.

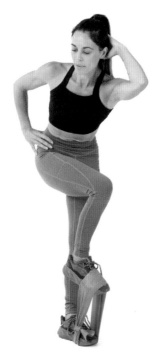

SUMO LATERAL CRUNCH

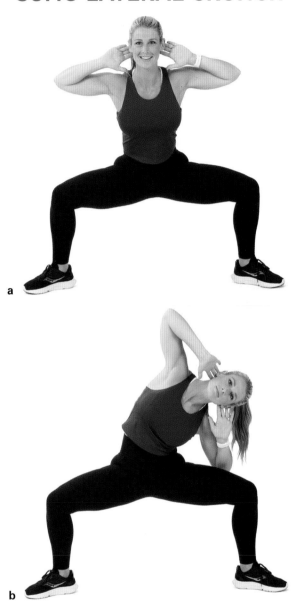

a

b

How It's Done

1. Stand in a sumo squat position with the feet in a wide stance (wider than shoulder-width apart); the toes and knees are turned out at about a 45-degree angle. With the chest lifted and proud, the shoulders back, and the hips aligned under the shoulders, lift through the arches of the feet, and bend the knees toward a 90-degree angle.

2. Place both hands behind the head with the fingers spread wide, thumbs at the nape of neck, and elbows wide.

3. As you exhale, bend the torso to one side, reaching the elbow toward the same-side thigh.
4. As you inhale and keep the abs engaged, lift the torso to return to the starting position.
5. Repeat for repetitions or switch sides.

Regressions and Progressions

1. Decrease the range of motion by standing more upright.
2. Increase the range of motion by deepening the sumo squat.

Safety Cues

1. Keep the shoulders back, chest lifted and proud, and knees back the entire time.
2. Keep the hips solid; control the pelvis, resisting the urge to rock or lift the hip to reach the elbow.

Variations

1. Extend the arm, and reach for the outside of the ankle in the crunch for deeper lateral flexion.
2. With a resistance band around the wrists, extend the arms overhead for more stability and shoulder challenge.

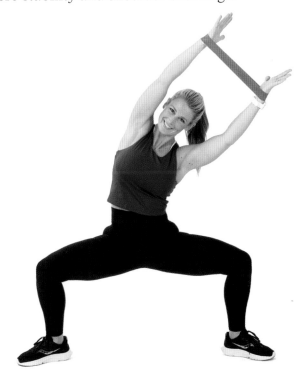

SUMO TWIST

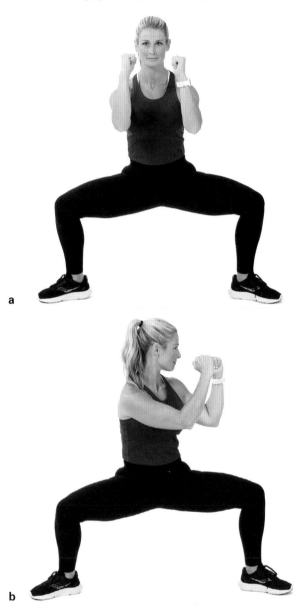

a

b

How It's Done

1. Stand in a sumo squat position with the feet in a wide stance (wider than shoulder-width apart) and the toes and knees diagonally turned out at about a 45-degree angle. With the chest lifted and proud, the shoulders back, and the hips aligned under the shoulders, lift through the arches of the feet, and bend the knees toward a 90-degree angle.

2. Bend the elbows at a 90-degree angle and in front of the chest. Make a fist like a boxer's guard.

3. As you exhale, twist the torso, moving one shoulder back and the other forward.

4. As you inhale, return the torso to center.

5. Repeat for repetitions or switch sides.

Regressions and Progressions

1. Stand more upright, and lessen the twist for a regression.

2. For a progression, sink deeper into the sumo squat, and twist farther for greater range of motion.

Safety Cues

1. Keep the shoulders back, chest lifted and proud, eyes focused forward, and knees back the entire time.

2. Keep the hips solid and controlled; resist the urge to rock the hips or bring the knees inward while twisting.

Variations

1. Slow down the exercise for added control, to help keep body alignment, and to prevent dizziness.

2. Add wrist weights for additional abdominal and shoulder muscle challenge.

3. Use a resistance band around the wrists, extending the arms in front of the torso for more stability and shoulder challenge.

4. Hold a medicine ball in front of the torso (with arms in or extended) for more abdominal challenge.

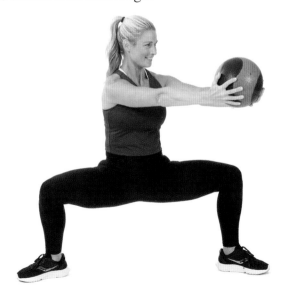

ANTERIOR PELVIC TILT

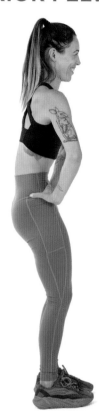

How It's Done

1. Stand tall in a neutral pelvis position with the shoulders back, chest up, abs braced, and a deep bend in both knees for a stable base. The toes and knees face forward, and the hands are placed on the hips.

2. As you exhale, relax the glutes and engage the abs, lifting the navel in and up; the bottom of the pelvis will rock forward.

3. As you inhale, relax the muscles and return to neutral pelvis.

4. Repeat for repetitions.

Regressions and Progressions

1. Perform a smaller pelvic movement but with long spine and optimal posture.
2. Take a bigger exhalation, and create greater pelvic tilt with a long spine.

Safety Cues

1. This is a small movement, so don't do a crunch; the shoulders remain back and down. Isolate the pelvis, and roll the navel in and up.
2. Relax the glutes, and engage the abs.
3. Use your breath to activate and engage the abs.
4. Be mindful that the exercise does not include a posterior pelvic tilt; always return to neutral pelvis alignment.

Variations

1. Deepen the knee bend for bigger movement.
2. Use a yoga strap around the mid back, and extend the arms in front to help set posture points.

SIDE HIP TUCK

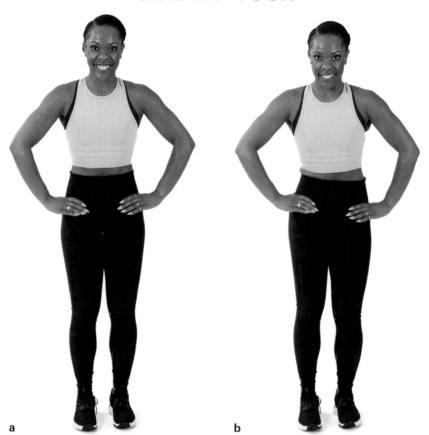

a   b

How It's Done

1. Stand tall with the pelvis neutral, shoulders back, chest up, and abs engaged, and deeply bend both knees for a stable base. The toes and knees are parallel and forward, and the hands are placed on the hips.

2. Keep both feet and heels connected with the ground.

3. As you exhale, engage the oblique abdominal muscles to lift the same-side hip to the side and up; the pelvis will rock forward.

4. As you inhale, return to neutral pelvis.

5. Repeat for repetitions or switch sides.

Regressions and Progressions

1. Perform smaller hip movements but with optimal spinal alignment and posture.
2. Take a bigger exhalation, and create greater hip lift with a long spine.

Safety Cues

1. Keep both feet planted on the ground; resist lifting the heel in order to lift the hip.
2. This is a small movement, so avoid crunching; the shoulders remain back and down. Isolate the pelvis, and roll the navel in and up.
3. Use your breath to activate and engage the abs.
4. Be mindful that there is no anterior or posterior pelvic tilt in the exercise; always return to neutral spinal and pelvic alignment.

Variations

1. Deepen the knee bend for bigger movement.
2. Use a yoga strap around the mid back with the arms extended in front to help set posture points.

ABS

CHAPTER 6

Floor and Seated Core Exercises

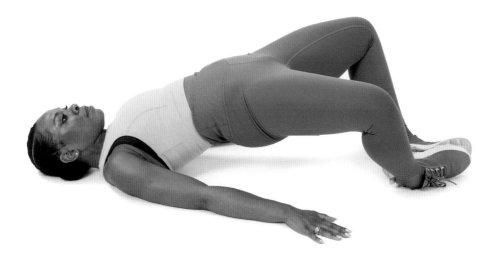

Training your glutes and abs in various positions and planes of motion will challenge your mind–body connection and improve your daily functional movements, such as turning around, picking yourself up from the floor, and moving side to side. The exercises in this chapter will help train your glutes and abs while also adding extra posture training for your back.

This book has established the benefits of exercising your core muscles; this chapter continues to define various ways of doing so. The floor-based exercises in this chapter may feel more accessible for some people because they require less balance challenge or less work against gravity compared to some exercises performed standing.

Be sure that your floor surface is clean and dry. Carpet and cushioned floors are great for these exercises. If you are exercising on a hard floor surface, an exercise mat is encouraged.

INCLINE GLUTE BRIDGE

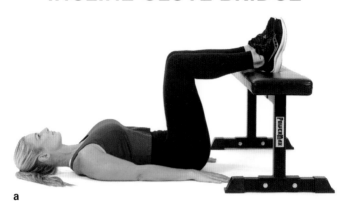

a

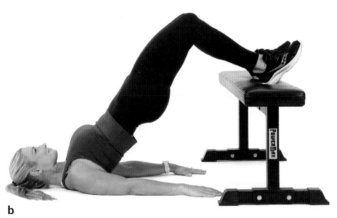

b

How It's Done

1. Lie supine (on your back) with the knees bent at 90 degrees. Relax the head, neck, and shoulders on the floor.

2. Place the heels of both feet on a stable, lifted, flat surface, such as a box or weight bench. The feet should be hip-width apart, and you should not feel pain in the knees.

3. Extend the arms along the sides of the torso with palms facing down.

4. Drive up through the heels to lift the glutes off the ground. Engage the glutes through this motion, keeping the navel drawn in and up. All of your weight should be balanced between the backs of the arms and the feet.

5. Make sure you lift the hips straight up and that the knees remain aligned with the hips and toes.

6. Return to the starting position by lowering the hips down with control and softly landing on the floor.
7. Repeat for repetitions.

Regressions and Progressions
1. To lessen the challenge, move the feet from an elevated surface to be flat on the ground, at the same level as the hips on the floor.
2. Add a barbell or resistance band at the front of the hips to increase muscular challenge.

Safety Cues
1. If you experience pain in the knees, try stepping the feet farther away from the glutes to increase the angle in the knee joints.
2. The head, neck, and shoulders should remain relaxed on the floor while performing this exercise to avoid straining the neck or back.

Variations
1. Raise the heels a few inches off of an elevated surface, balancing on the balls of the feet (as in relevé).
2. Wear a resistance band around the thighs (the area above the knees and below the hips) and open knees outward for an added abduction on the concentric phase of the exercise (on the way up; see photo on this page).
3. Wear a resistance band across the hips, holding it under the palms for added resistance on the way up.

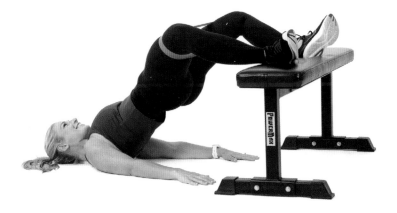

DECLINE HIP BRIDGE

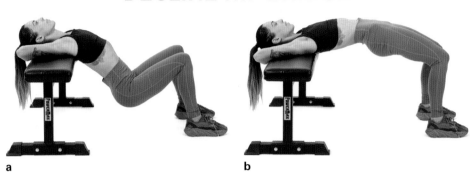

a   b

How It's Done

1. Rest the upper back and shoulders on a bench, and keep the spine neutral from head to hips; the knees are bent, and the feet are flat on the floor.
2. Place the palms behind the head or at the hips.
3. Drive the hips up by pressing through the heels. Engage the glutes through this motion, and keep the navel drawn in and up. All of your weight should be balanced between the feet, the middle of the back, and the shoulders.
4. Make sure you lift the hips straight up and that the knees remain aligned with the hips and toes. The body is parallel to the floor.
5. Lower the hips to return to the starting position.
6. Repeat for repetitions.

Regressions and Progressions

1. Take the torso to flat ground, and perform the exercise completely on the floor.
2. Hold a barbell at the hips for added resistance to progress this move.

Safety Cues

1. Keep the mid back and the backs of the shoulders on the bench. While pressing the hips up, the head should relax on the bench surface.
2. Keep the head and spine aligned, looking directly up.
3. The feet should remain aligned with the hips throughout the exercise.

Variations

1. See the Regressions and Progressions section of this exercise for additional variations.
2. Wear a band around the thighs for an added abduction on the concentric phase of the exercise.

HIP ABDUCTION

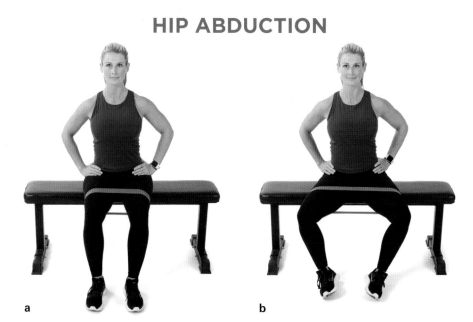

a

b

How It's Done

1. Sit tall on a bench or chair with the ankles aligned under the knees, the knees hip-width apart, and a resistance band around the thighs.
2. Press the knees outward in a controlled motion, keeping the feet relatively in place; the feet may supinate or roll out.
3. Keep tension in the resistance band as you slowly bring the knees back in toward the midline of the body.
4. Repeat for repetitions.

Regressions and Progressions

1. Shorten the range of motion or distance that the knees move outward for a regression.
2. For a progression, increase the resistance level on the band for added challenge.

Safety Cues

1. Maintain an upright position, keeping the abs engaged and shoulders back.
2. Do not rush the movement; work in a controlled manner.
3. Wear the resistance band above the knees and not on the knees.

Variations

1. This exercise can be performed without a band, but you must cognitively focus on glute engagement and activation to abduct the hips, opening the knees outward.
2. Use a seated abduction machine for greater weight selection and resistance level.

KNEELING KICKBACK

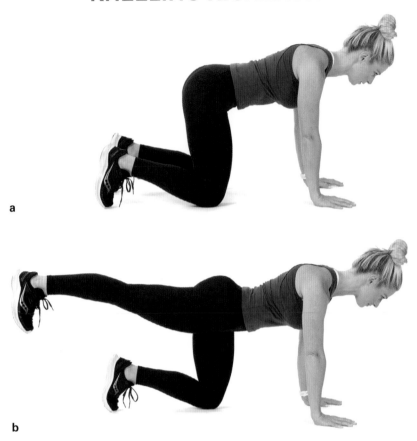

a

b

How It's Done

1. Begin on all fours, aligning the hands directly under the shoulders and the knees under the hips.
2. Dorsiflex at the ankles.
3. Extend one leg by pressing one foot back and up, lifting the knee and ankle to align at hip height.
4. With control, lower the knee back down to the starting position.
5. Repeat for repetitions or switch sides.

Regressions and Progressions

1. Decrease the height of the leg on the lift to avoid pinching in the lower back to regress the exercise.
2. Add a resistance band under the bottom of the foot with handles anchored under the palms for more muscular challenge.

Safety Cues

1. Keep the spine long, and avoid dipping or sagging in the lower back and shoulders.
2. Work to steady the hips and keep the abs engaged throughout the exercise.
3. Press the floor away with the arms, and keep the shoulders away from the ears.

Variations

1. Perform this exercise on the forearms or palms with arms extended.
2. Use a resistance band around the arches of both feet to intensify the exercise.

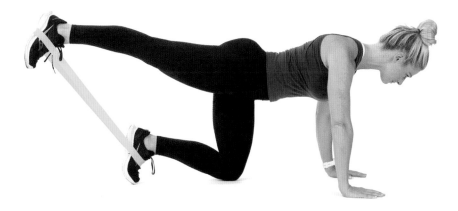

GLUTES

KNEELING HIP THRUSTER

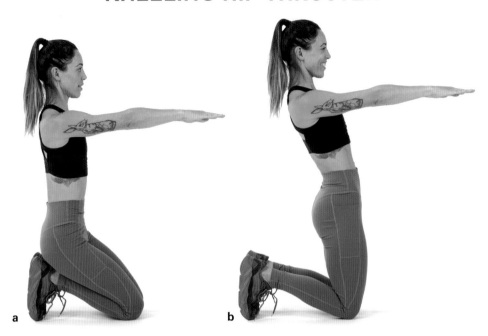

a   b

How It's Done

1. Start by sitting upright in a kneeling position with the toes tucked under and the arms extended in front of the torso at shoulder height.
2. Sit on the heels, engage the glutes, then lift your body up, extending the hips to stand on the knees.
3. Slowly, with control, lower the hips to sit on the heels.
4. Repeat for repetitions.

Regressions and Progressions

1. Hold a weighted fitness bar or barbell in front of you to add a third leg to help with balance.
2. Pulling some form of resistance from behind will create more resistance to increase work for the glutes.

Safety Cues

Avoid hyperextending the low back; do not press the hips so far forward that you feel pain in the low back.

Variations

1. Foot placement is optional. The feet can be parallel, or the toes can be together to create a triangle with the legs.

2. Place resistance tubing or cable handles at the hips with a partner being the anchor point behind you holding the tubing handles on the ground to create resistance on the hip thrust.

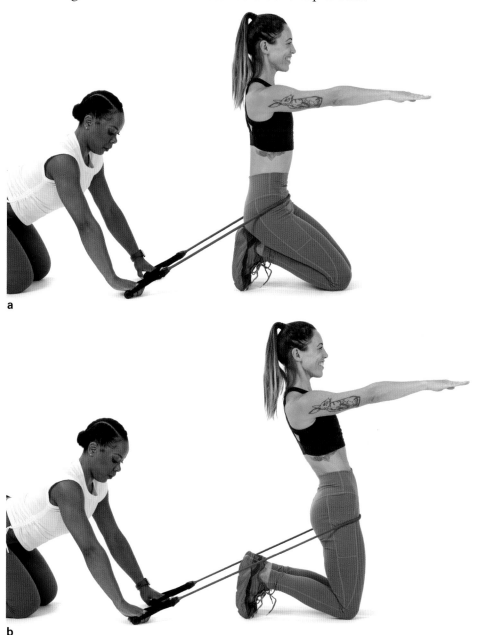

a

b

BRIDGE WITH KNEE ABDUCTION

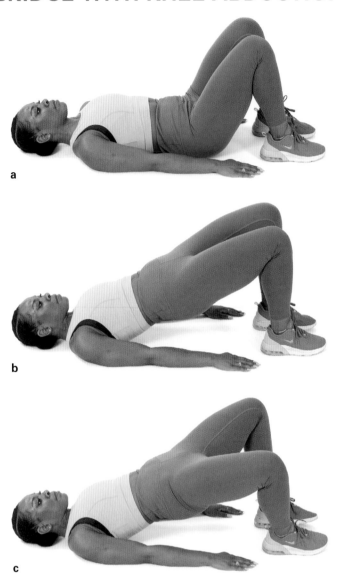

a

b

c

How It's Done

1. Start by lying supine with the knees bent and the feet flat on the floor. The feet and knees should be about hip-distance apart.

2. Relax the head, neck, and shoulders, and place the hands alongside the torso, palm-side down on the floor.

3. Activate the glutes as you push through the heels and lift the hips straight up. Your body should be straight in a diagonal line from shoulders to knees.

4. At the peak of the hip bridge, open the knees out to the sides, squeezing the glutes.
5. Close the knees back toward the midline of your body.
6. Lower the hips slowly, returning to the starting position.
7. Repeat for repetitions.

Regressions and Progressions

1. Decrease the range of motion and how high you lift the hips, but continue to activate the glutes on the lift.
2. Hold a barbell at the front of the hips to create an additional muscular challenge.

Safety Cues

1. You should not feel aches or pains in the knees. If you do, step both feet away from the glutes for more distance between the heels and butt.
2. Avoid lifting the hips so high that you feel tightness in the low back. If you feel pain in the low back as you lift the hips, perhaps you have lifted too high.
3. If using a resistance band, keep tension in the band the entire time.

Variations

Wrap a resistance band around the thighs, and press against the resistance of the band during the abduction phase to create tension. Be sure to wear the band flat around the thighs; it should be above the knees and not on the knees.

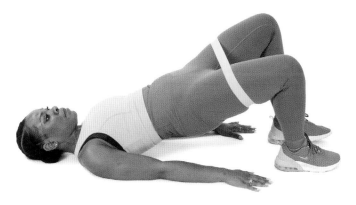

FIRE HYDRANT

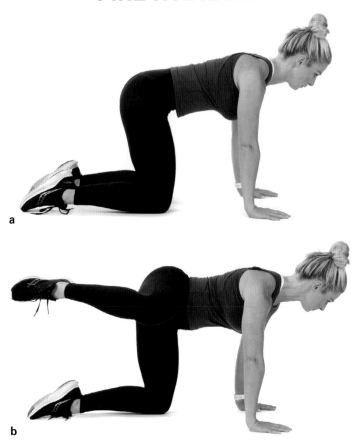

a

b

How It's Done

1. Begin on all fours, aligning the hands directly under the shoulders and the knees under the hips.
2. Brace the abs, and engage the glutes.
3. Keep the torso and pelvis stable as you laterally move one leg so that the knee opens out and the inner thigh is parallel to the floor.
4. Contract the thigh as you lower the leg back to the starting position.
5. Repeat for repetitions or switch sides.

Regressions and Progressions

1. Shorten the range of motion of the leg lift to lessen the challenge.
2. Keep a long spine, but lower from the palms to the forearms to stabilize the setup.
3. Wrap a band around the thighs for more muscular challenge to the glutes.

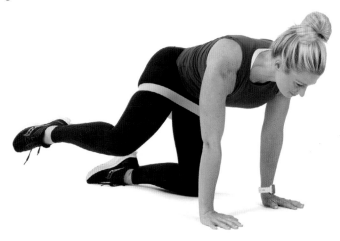

Safety Cues

1. Keep the spine long, abs activated, and glutes engaged the entire time.
2. Keep the hips aligned with the shoulders.
3. To prevent knee pain, you can put something soft under the knees for extra cushion.
4. Avoid dipping in the low back or lifting one hip higher than the other.

Variations

See the Regressions and Progressions section of this exercise for variations.

GLUTES

SINGLE-LEG BRIDGE

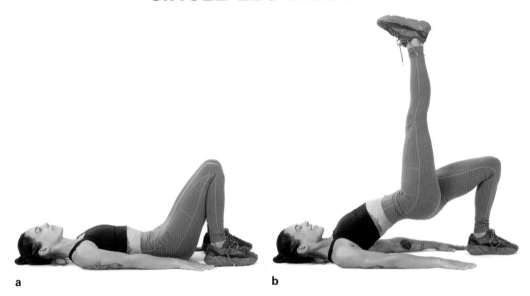

a   b

How It's Done

1. Start by lying in a supine position with the palms down, knees comfortably bent, and feet hip-width apart and flat on the floor.
2. Press the feet firmly into the floor. Activate the glutes, extend one leg in the air, press the opposite foot into the floor, and lift the hips up.
3. With control, slowly lower the hips down to the floor while keeping the leg extended.
4. Repeat for repetitions or switch sides, starting from step 2.

Regressions and Progressions

1. To lessen the challenge, do a standard hip bridge with both feet on the floor.
2. Lift the heels (relevé position instead of flatfoot position) for an added challenge.

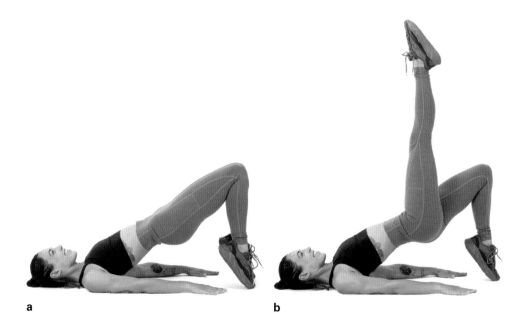

a   b

Safety Cues

1. You should not feel aches or pains in the knees. If you do, step the feet away from the glutes for more distance between the heels and butt.

2. You should not lift the hips so high that you feel tightness in the low back. If you feel pain in the low back as you lift the hips, perhaps you have lifted too high.

3. If using a resistance band, keep tension in the band the entire time.

Variations

1. See the Regressions and Progressions section of this exercise for additional variations.

2. Add weight or some form of resistance at the front of the hips to increase muscular challenge.

3. Try wearing a resistance band around the thighs and adding an abduction on the concentric phase of the exercise.

4. Anchor a resistance band across the hips while holding it under the palms to add resistance on the way up.

BUTTERFLY HIP LIFT

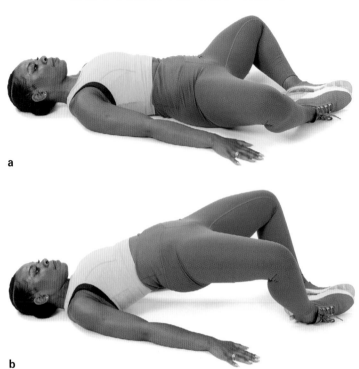

a

b

How It's Done

1. Start by lying supine with the palms down, the knees comfortably bent, and the feet flat on the floor.
2. Separate the knees outward as far as they will comfortably open. You will feel a slight stretch in the inner thighs.
3. Bring the soles of the feet together, and activate the glutes.
4. Pressing the sides of the feet into the floor, lift the hips up. Your body should form a straight line from the shoulders all the way to the pelvis.
5. Balance on the backs of the shoulders.
6. With control, slowly lower the hips.
7. Repeat for repetitions starting with step 4.

Regressions and Progressions

1. A regressive option is to keep your knees together or not open them as wide.
2. A progression is to gently add resistance at the front of your hips to make this move more glute intensive.

Safety Cues

1. Be sure the spine remains long from the neck to tailbone.
2. Pay attention to how the hips and knees respond to this move. It should not cause pain in the joints.

Variations

1. Wear a band around the thighs to create tension on the abduction.
2. Anchor a resistance band across the hips while holding it under the palms to add resistance on the way up.

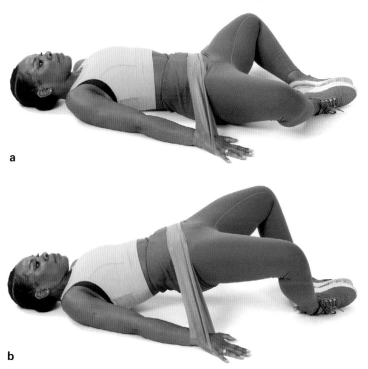

a

b

DONKEY KICK

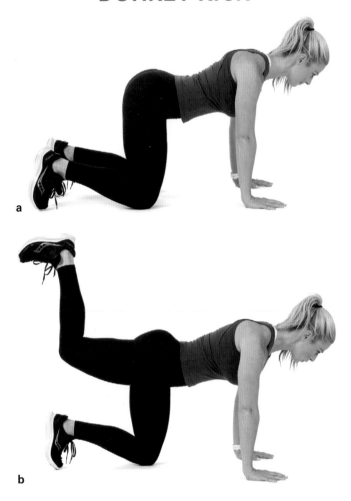

a

b

How It's Done

1. Begin on all fours, aligning the hands directly under the shoulders and the knees under the hips.
2. Brace the abs and engage the glutes to keep the torso and pelvis stable.
3. Keeping both knees bent, lead with the sole of one foot and lift it toward the sky; the thigh should be parallel to the floor.
4. Lower the knee, returning to the starting position.
5. Repeat for repetitions or switch sides.

Regressions and Progressions

1. Shortening your range of motion or coming down onto your forearms are optional regressions.
2. Wear a band around the thighs to add tension and resistance.
3. Secure a dumbbell behind the lifted knee by closing the calf toward the thigh to increase the glute challenge.

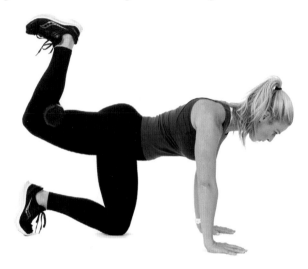

Safety Cues

1. Keep the spine long, abs activated, and glutes engaged the entire time.
2. Keep the hips aligned with the shoulders.
3. Use something soft under the knees for extra cushion.
4. Avoid dipping in the low back or lifting one hip higher than the other.

Variations

1. See the regressions and progressions section of this exercise for optimal variations.
2. Try using machines for this exercise. Some gyms have pin-select glute machines that you can use for performing this exercise and adding additional weight resistance.

FROGGER

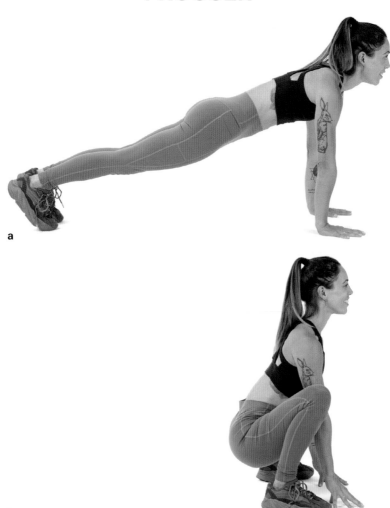

a

b

How It's Done

1. Begin in a plank position, with the palms on the floor directly under the shoulders, the legs long, and the feet about hip-width apart. Your body should be in one long line from the crown of the head to the soles of the feet.
2. Step or jump the feet forward, leaping like a frog; land with the knees bent and the feet on the outsides of the bent elbows.
3. Land with the hips low in a squatting position.
4. Engaging the glutes, jump the feet back and land on the balls of the feet in the starting plank position.
5. Repeat for repetitions.

Regressions and Progressions

1. A regression is to walk the feet in and out instead of jumping.
2. A progression is to spring-load the weight back into the glutes before jumping the feet forward. To do this move, start in plank. Then, bend the knees as you push the hips back over the heels, push out with a jump, catch hang time in the air, and land the feet wide outside the elbows.

Safety Cues

Be sure to broadly jump and land softly on the feet with bent elbows and knees to protect the joints.

Variations

Wear a resistance band around the thighs, high above the knees, for added muscular conditioning.

GLUTES

EXTENDED REVERSE LEG LIFT

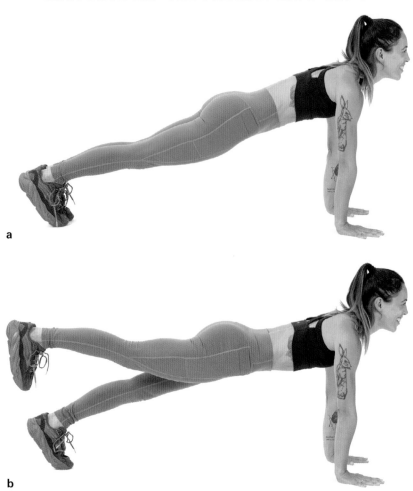

a

b

How It's Done

1. Begin in a plank position, with the palms on the floor directly under the shoulders and the legs long. Your body should be in one long line from the crown of the head to the soles of the feet.
2. Engaging the glutes and leading with the heel of each foot, lift and lower one leg at a time.
3. For each repetition, contract the glute muscles at the top of the leg lift, release the contraction, then lower the leg back down to the starting position.
4. Repeat for repetitions or switch sides.

Regressions and Progressions

1. To regress this move, begin in an all-fours position instead of a plank.
2. Wear a resistance band around the thighs or use ankle weights for added resistance.

Safety Cues

1. Joints should not be locked in plank position; instead, muscles should be firmly engaged.
2. Avoid dipping the low back on the leg lifts. Keep the spine long and stable. If your low back sags on the leg lift, it may mean that you are lifting the leg too high.

Variations

See the Regressions and Progressions section of this exercise for variations.

CLAM

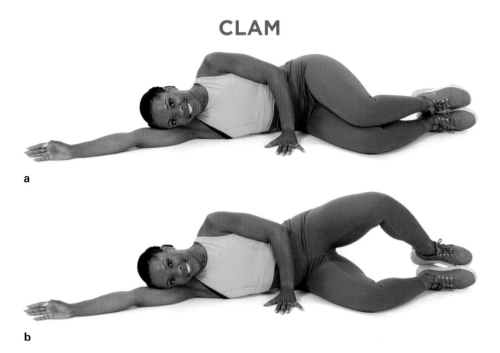

a

b

How It's Done

1. Start in a side-lying position, with the bottom arm extended on the floor and the head resting on the arm. The hips, legs, and feet are stacked and the knees are bent at a 90-degree angle.
2. Place the top hand on the floor in front of the navel to stabilize the torso.
3. Keeping the bottom leg on the floor and activating the glutes, lift the top knee away from the bottom knee as if opening a clamshell. You should feel the tops and outer edges of the glutes engaged.
4. Lower the top knee to the starting position.
5. Repeat for repetitions or switch sides.

Regressions and Progressions

1. Arm placement is optional, based on comfort and preference. You can support your head on the arm or in the hand with a bent elbow for comfort to the neck.
2. You can prop yourself on the forearm as a progressive option that challenges the obliques.

Safety Cues

1. Be sure that the hip bones are stacked.
2. Brace the abs to stabilize the pelvis and torso during this movement.

Variations

Wear a resistance band around the thighs for more glute activation. Keep the band above the knees, and keep tension in the band the entire time.

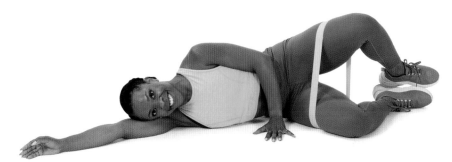

SEAL HEEL CLAP

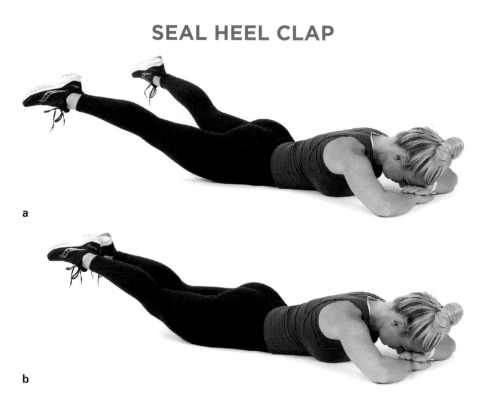

a

b

How It's Done

1. Start in a prone position (lying flat on your abdomen), with the legs extended behind you. Fold the arms, and rest the forehead on the forearms.

2. As you exhale, engage the thighs, glutes, and back muscles, lifting the heels up and thighs off of the floor. Keep the legs extended long behind you.

3. Once the thighs are lifted from the floor, start clapping or beating the heels together while they are suspended in the air.

4. Keep clapping the heels together for a number of repetitions or until you feel the burn in the glutes.

5. Disconnect the heels, then lower the thighs and feet to the starting position.

6. Repeat for repetitions.

Regressions and Progressions

1. For a regression, lessen the range of motion when lifting the legs away from the floor.
2. For a progression, stabilize on your forearms and palms by pushing the forearms and palms deeper into the floor as you lift the chest completely off the floor for a back extension.

Safety Cues

1. Keep the spine long.
2. Keep the forehead in contact with your forearms.
3. Lift the legs using the glutes and thigh muscles and not the low back.

Variations

1. Loop a resistance band around the thighs or just above the ankles to add to the glute challenge on the abduction.
2. Wear ankle weights for added resistance and muscular challenge.

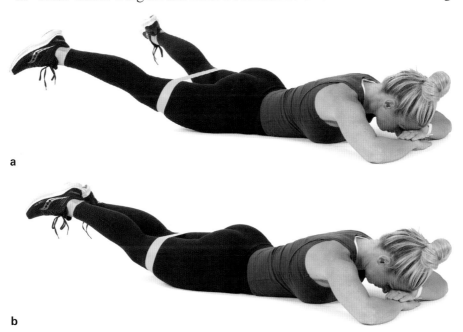

a

b

ABS

FORWARD CRUNCH

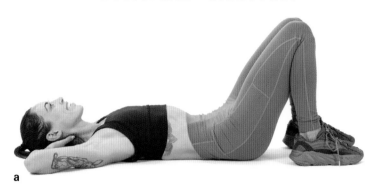

a

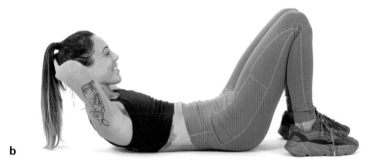

b

How It's Done

1. Lie supine with the knees bent and the feet flat on the floor.
2. Place the hands gently behind the head; avoid pulling on the back of the head or neck.
3. As you exhale and contract the abs, lift the shoulder blades from the floor. The mid to low back remains on the floor; this is a crunch and not a full sit-up.
4. As you inhale, lower the upper back and head to the starting position.
5. Repeat for repetitions.

Regressions and Progressions
1. Shortening the lift is a regression.
2. Lifting higher to a full sit-up is a progression.

Safety Cues
1. Avoid tugging or yanking on your neck on the crunch.
2. Keep a light, featherlight touch at the nape of your neck.
3. Keep your chin lifted, and avoid tucking it to your chest.

Variations
1. Place the arms across the chest instead of the hands behind the head.
2. Lift the legs to progress the exercise or alleviate tension in the back.
3. Place a small exercise ball at the small of the back to increase range of motion when performing the crunch.

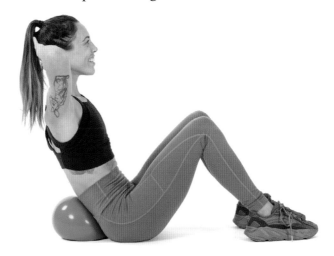

SIDE CRUNCH

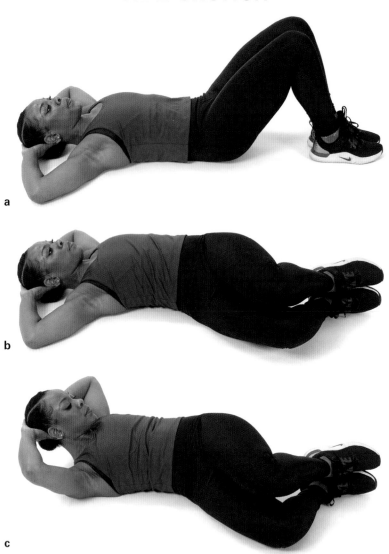

a

b

c

How It's Done

1. Lie supine with the knees bent and the feet flat on the floor.
2. Place the hands gently behind the head; avoid pulling on the back of the head or neck.
3. Twist from the waist to move both legs to one side, stacked on top of each other. The chest remains up toward the ceiling.
4. As you exhale and contract the abs, lift the shoulder blades from the floor. The low back can remain on the floor; this is a crunch and not a full sit-up.
5. As you inhale, slowly lower the upper back and head to the starting position.
6. Repeat for repetitions or switch sides.

Regressions and Progressions

1. Decreasing range of motion is a regression.
2. Increasing range of motion by crunching deeper and lifting the head, neck, and shoulders higher off the floor is a progression.

Safety Cues

1. You should not experience any strain on the back when performing this exercise. Ensure both legs fall over to the same side by twisting at the waist.
2. Avoid tugging or yanking on the neck during the crunch.
3. Keep a light, featherlight touch at the nape of the neck.
4. Keep the chin lifted, and avoid tucking it to the chest.

Variations

1. Place the arms across the chest instead of the hands behind the head.
2. Hold a weighted plate at the chest to make the exercise more challenging.

ABS

V-SIT

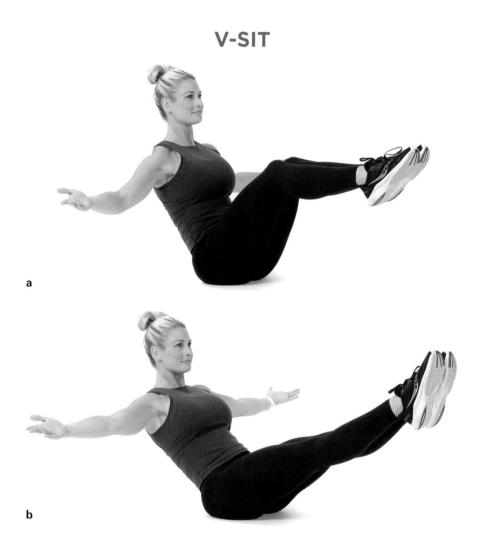

a

b

How It's Done

1. Start balancing on the sit bones with the knees bent, chest open, shoulders back, arms reaching out to the sides, and legs and feet hovering off the floor; this position is similar to a boat pose in yoga.

2. Extend the legs out long and hinge the hips back to open out from the boat pose position.

3. Engage the core muscles to tuck the legs back in, returning to the starting position.

4. Repeat for repetitions.

Regressions and Progressions

1. A regression can be to place your hands on the floor to your sides.
2. For an additional regression, extend one leg at a time.
3. Extend your arms overhead and legs long to add challenge to the exercise.

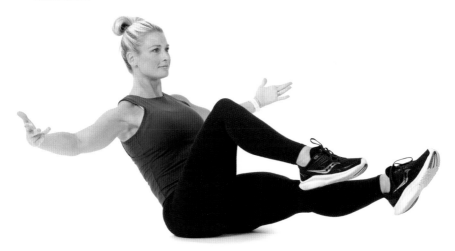

Safety Cues

Avoid overcompensating with the hip flexors. If you feel fatigue in the hip flexors, shorten the range of motion or take a break.

Variations

1. Place a small exercise ball at the small of your back for added support.
2. Hold a weighted ball in either hand, or between both hands with arms extended overhead, to intensify the abdominal challenge.

K-CRUNCH

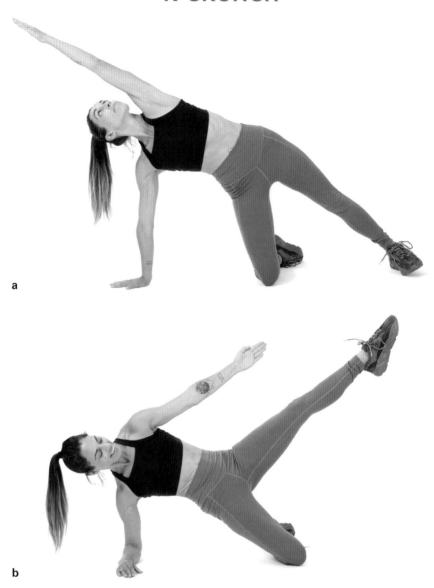

a

b

How It's Done

1. Kneel on one knee with the same side palm down and the other leg extended; the active arm and leg are extended. Your body forms the letter K.
2. Move the active arm and leg in toward one another; this action is the crunch.
3. With control, extend the active limbs back out to the starting position.
4. Repeat for repetitions or switch sides.

Regressions and Progressions

1. Bend the elbow and knee to lessen the challenge.
2. Lower to the forearm for less balance challenge, as seen in photo *b* for this exercise.
3. Extend the arm and leg for greater reach, or extend the bottom leg into a full side plank for added effort.

Safety Cues

1. Be sure to keep a long neck and avoid crunching the ear to the shoulder.
2. Avoid locking the elbow, which can cause undue stress on the joint.

Variations

1. See the Regressions and Progressions section of this exercise for additional variations.
2. Hold a light dumbbell in the active hand to add muscular resistance and challenge.

KNEELING TORSO TWIST

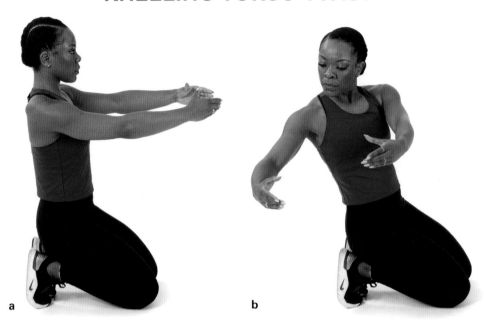

a   b

How It's Done

1. Start in a kneeling position, sitting back on the heels with the toes pressing into the floor.
2. Extend the arms out in front of you, then rotate the torso to one side.
3. Twist as far back behind you as you can go, return the torso to face forward, then twist to the other side; imagine connecting the dots from front, to side, to front, to the other side, and so on.
4. Repeat for repetitions.

Regressions and Progressions

1. Regress the exercise by reaching only one arm at a time back as you twist.
2. Another regression is to shorten the lever of the arms, crossing the arms at the chest on the twist.
3. A progression is to increase your range of motion by twisting deeper and reaching farther back.

Safety Cues

1. Keep the core muscles engaged, and utilize your inhalations and exhalations to aid in the deep twist.
2. A nice stretching feeling comes with the twist, but you should not feel straining. If so, you have twisted too far back.

Variations

1. Twist back; as you untwist to face forward, sit up off of the heels for added abdominal and glute work.
2. Holding a medicine ball, twist back and place the ball behind you. Twist to the other side to pick up the ball. Repeat the cycle for as many repetitions as you choose, then switch leading directions.

ABS

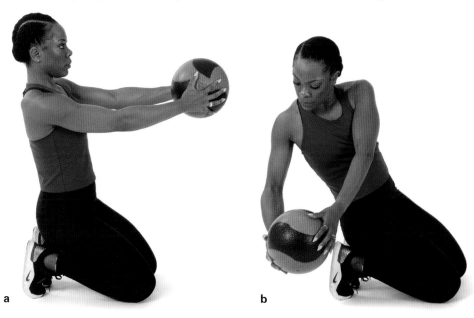

a   b

ABDOMINAL PUSHOUT

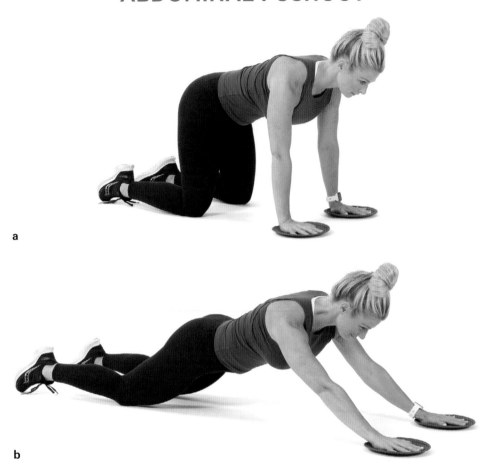

a

b

How It's Done

1. Start on all fours with a glider under each hand.
2. While contracting the abs and back and stabilizing the hips, push the arms forward; this action is the pushout.
3. Push out as far as you can go while maintaining core engagement and while keeping the hips and shoulders aligned; allow no sagging in the hips or belly.
4. Contracting the muscles of the torso, smoothly pull the arms back in to the starting position.
5. Repeat for repetitions.

Regressions and Progressions

1. Shorten the distance gliding out or extend one arm at a time for a regression.
2. A progression is to lengthen and extend your reach, reaching farther out as you glide.

Safety Cues

1. Avoid pushing too far out; it can require jerky or popping movements to pull back in.
2. If the shoulders are bothering you, shorten the distance on the pushout.
3. Avoid sagging in the low back when performing this move; position yourself in a long, plank-like position with one long line from the crown of the head to the tailbone.
4. Place a folded mat or other cushion under the knees for comfort.

Variations

1. Try directional changes on the pushout to add challenge and variety.
2. In addition to gliders, you can use a towel or ab roller to perform this exercise.

PILATES ROLL-UP

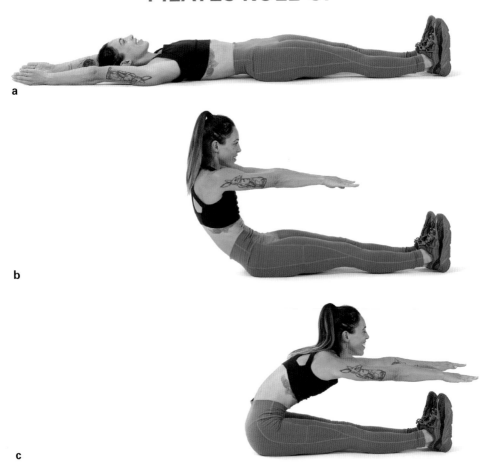

a

b

c

How It's Done

1. Start by lying in a supine position with the thighs squeezed together, the legs flat and straight on the floor, and the arms extended over the head.

2. Brace the abs, making them taut. The muscles you are focusing on are the pelvic floor muscles that engage when you let out a big laugh and when you try to stop yourself from urinating.

3. Rock the pelvis up and in, scoop the navel in, pull the abs in deep, and depress the low back even more toward the floor.

4. Still able to breathe deeply (not holding your breath), keep this ab and thigh engagement.

5. As you forcibly exhale, gradually peel the upper body off the ground in a smooth motion. Start with the arms, adding a C-curve in the spine, and curl the body up and over the legs; tuck the chin on the way up, and reach for the toes.

6. As you inhale, reverse this smooth motion with control; maintain the C-curve as you gradually lower to the starting position.

7. Repeat for repetitions.

Regressions and Progressions

1. Ideally the legs remain extended throughout this move, but bent knees are acceptable to release tension in the back and the backs of the legs.

2. If you get stuck rolling up or down, using an elbow as a kickstand to push off is a regression option.

3. For a progression, squeeze a prop in between the hands to adduct more chest muscles and to increase concentration on core contraction.

Safety Cues

1. Move with a deep breath; move slowly with muscular control and not momentum.

2. Focus on the C-curve of the spine and the abdominal contraction.

3. This exercise requires good spinal flexibility and core strength. If at any time you experience pain in the neck or back, stop the exercise.

Variations

Try using a resistance ring, yoga block, or small exercise ball between the palms to add adducting resistance; it will recruit more chest muscles and add concentration on core contraction.

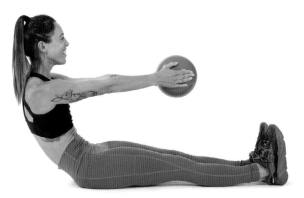

LATERAL ANKLE TOUCH

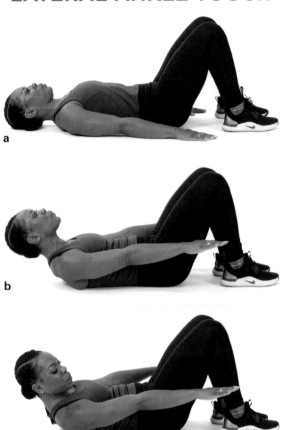

a

b

c

How It's Done

1. Start by lying in a supine position with the arms down to the sides, palms down, knees bent, and feet flat on the floor.

2. As you exhale, brace the abs, making them taut. You are focusing on the transverse abdominis muscles, the deep muscles that engage when you let out a big laugh or cough.

3. Rock the pelvis in and up, scooping the navel in and depressing the low back even more toward the floor.

4. Keeping this engagement in the abs, lift the head, neck, and shoulders off the floor; you are in an abdominal crunch.

5. Reach the fingertips of one hand toward the same-side ankle by doing an oblique crunch.

6. Return to center.

7. Repeat for repetitions or switch sides.

Regressions and Progressions

1. For a regression, slow the movement; relax the shoulders, neck, and head back down to the floor each time you return to center.
2. For a progression, lift the head, neck, and shoulder blades off the floor to form a deeper abdominal crunch.

Safety Cues

Come out of the exercise any time you feel tension or pain in the neck or back.

Variations

Lift your legs to a 90-degree angle in a supine tabletop or "dead bug" like position.

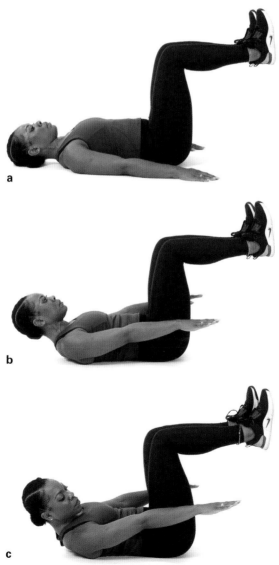

a

b

c

ABS

BICYCLE

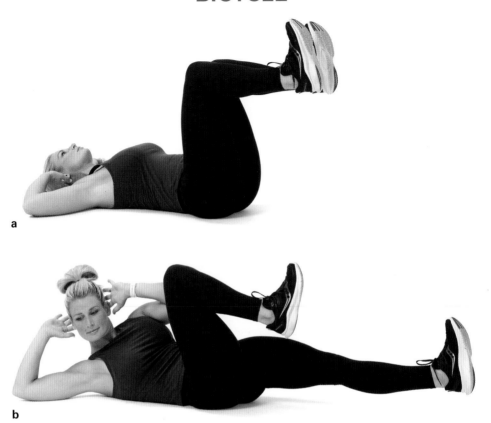

a

b

How It's Done

1. Lie in a supine position with the palms behind the head and the elbows wide. Lift the knees toward the chest, then bend them to a 90-degree angle and align them over the hips.
2. As you exhale, brace the abs and lift the head, neck, and shoulders to a crunch position.
3. Twisting the torso toward the right side, move the left shoulder toward the right knee as you extend the left leg out long.
4. Inhale to return to center, with both knees at a 90-degree angle.
5. Repeat for repetitions or switch sides.

Regressions and Progressions

1. A regression is to shorten the distance you extend the legs.
2. A progression is to extend the legs longer and lower to the floor for more abdominal challenge.

Safety Cues

1. Be sure to keep the back of your hips connected with the floor.
2. Relax the jaw, and relax the head into the hands to help alleviate neck tension.

Variations

Wear a resistance band around your shoes with the ankles dorsiflexed to add more abdominal challenge.

ABS

SIDE PLANK

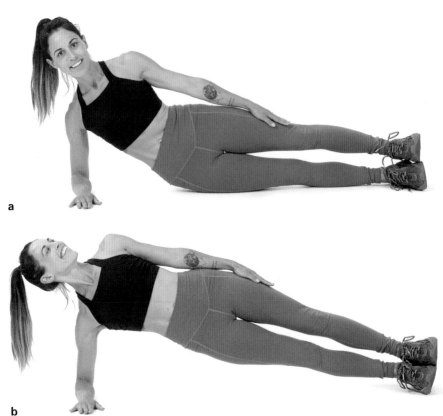

a

b

How It's Done

1. Start in a side-lying position with the bottom forearm on the floor; the elbow is bent at 90 degrees and aligned under the shoulder. The legs are sealed and stacked, and your body is in one long line. The top arm rests along the top side of the body.

2. As you exhale, while bracing the abs and lengthening the spine, push against the floor with the forearm and blade edge of the bottom foot, lifting the bottom hip off the floor. Keep your body in a long, straight line. Hold the position.

3. As you inhale, lower the hips back down to the floor and unbrace the abs.

4. Repeat for repetitions or switch sides.

Regressions and Progressions

1. A regression is to bend the bottom knee and pull the bottom foot behind you to create a kickstand of support for the side plank.
2. A progression is to lift the top leg and arm for a greater stability challenge.

Safety Cues

1. Keep the abs braced and active the entire time.
2. Find space between the ears and shoulders, not crunching in your neck. Think of long, straight spinal posture from the crown of the head all the way to the feet.

Variations

Try wearing a resistance band around the legs (just above the ankles) or around your shoes, then lift the top leg to increase muscular challenge. If using a resistance band, keep tension in the band the entire time.

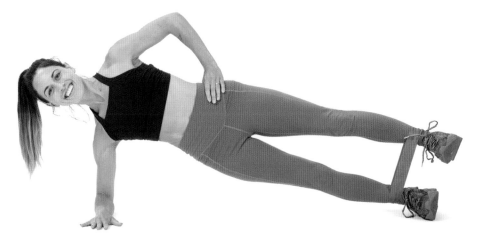

WINDSHIELD WIPER

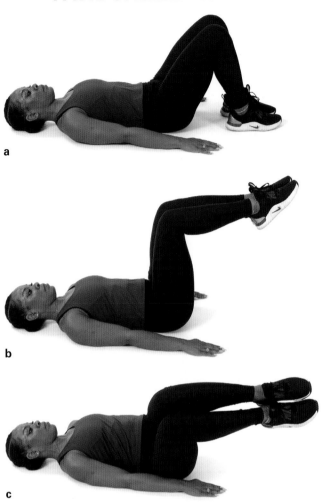

a

b

c

How It's Done

1. Start by lying in a supine position with the palms down, knees bent, and feet flat on the floor.

2. As you exhale, brace the abs, making them taut. You are focusing on the transverse abdominis muscles that engage when you let out a big laugh or cough.

3. Rock the pelvis in and up, scooping the navel in and depressing the low back even more toward the floor.

4. Lift the knees toward the chest, then bend them to a 90-degree angle and align them over the hips to a supine tabletop or "dead bug" like position.

5. Seal the thighs together, and stabilize the pelvis. The gaze is straight up.

6. Exhaling and moving with control, sweep both knees over to one side until you feel additional abdominal tension.
7. As you inhale, lift the knees back to center, aligning them over the hips.
8. Repeat steps 6 and 7 for repetitions or switch sides.

Regressions and Progressions

1. A regression is to not drop the knees as far down to the floor.
2. A progression is to seal the palms together in line with the chest, extending the arms and sweeping both arms to the opposite direction as the knees drop. Your gaze follows the sealed palms.

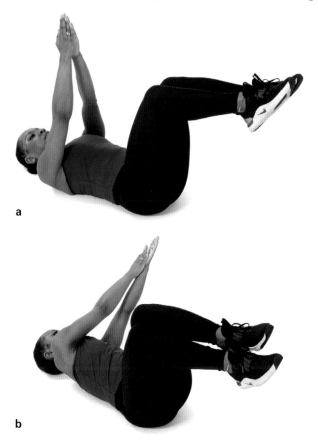

a

b

Safety Cues

Be sure to stabilize the spine and pelvis from the crown of the head to the tailbone before beginning the twist.

Variations

See the Regressions and Progressions section of this exercise for variations.

ABS

PLANK SAW

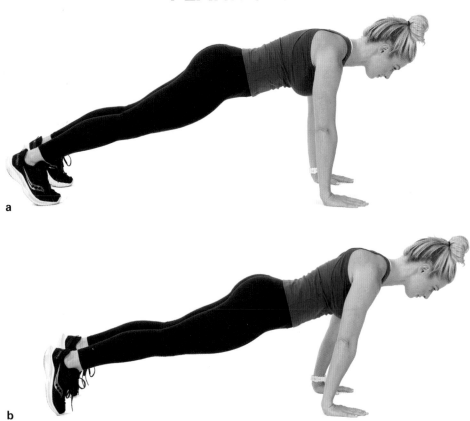

a

b

How It's Done

1. Begin in a prone position (on your belly) with the hands directly under the shoulders and the toes tucked under.

2. As you exhale, press the palms and toes firmly into the floor, pushing your body up to a full plank position. Your body is in a long line from the head to the heels.

3. As you inhale, shift your body forward until the nose is ahead of the fingertips, then shift back, making a sawing motion with your body.

4. Repeat for repetitions.

Regressions and Progressions

1. A regression is to perform this move on the forearms instead of on the palms.
2. A progression is to lift one leg at a time as you shift your body forward.

Safety Cues

Brace your abs and resist sagging in your lower back.

Variations

Place one glider under each hand. Shift your body forward as in the original exercise, and extend one arm and hand at a time by pushing forward and pulling back.

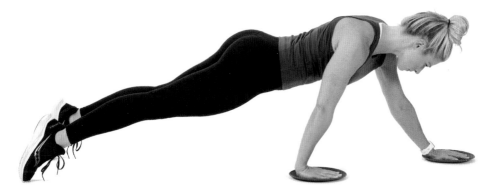

ABS

PLANK HIP DIP

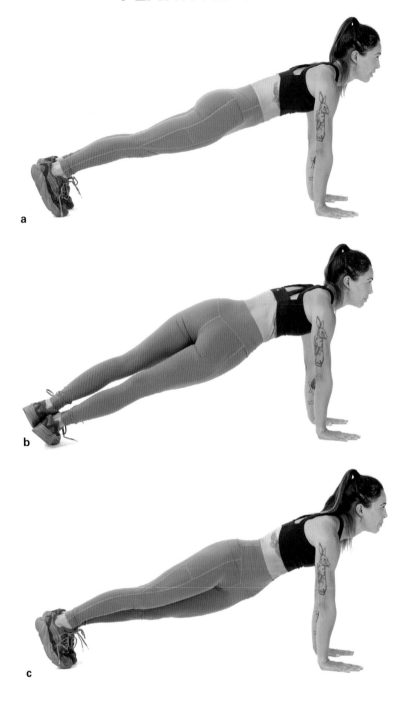

a

b

c

How It's Done

1. Begin in a prone position with the hands directly under the shoulders and the toes tucked under.
2. As you exhale, press the palms and toes firmly into the floor, pushing your body up to a full plank position. Your body is in a long line from the head to the heels.
3. Inhale and seal the thighs together, brace the abs firmly, and stabilize the pelvis.
4. On the exhale, in an arcing motion, tip the hips over to one side; keep both hands on the floor throughout this motion.
5. As you inhale, lift the hips back to center.
6. Repeat steps 4 and 5 for repetitions or switch sides.

Regressions and Progressions

1. A regression is to perform this move on the forearms instead of on the palms.
2. A progression is to wear a resistance band around the thighs or just above the ankles and keep the legs apart with tension on the band for more of a core challenge. If using a resistance band, keep tension in the band the entire time.

Safety Cues

1. Keep the spine long, hips stable, and abs engaged, and keep breathing deeply the entire time.
2. You should not have any sagging between the shoulder blades or in the hips while in plank position.

Variations

See the Regressions and Progressions section of this exercise for variations.

THREAD THE NEEDLE

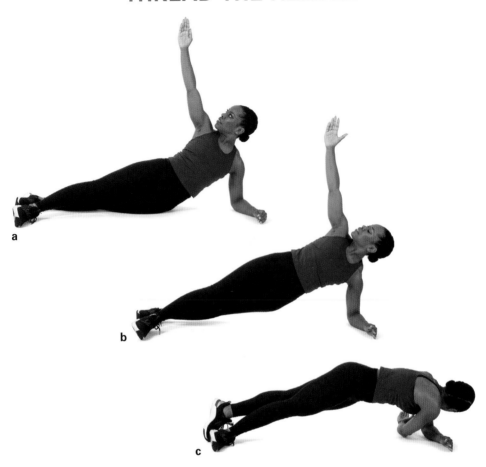

How It's Done

1. Start in a side-lying position with the bottom forearm on the floor; the elbow is bent at 90 degrees and aligned under the shoulder. The top arm is extended with the wrist aligned above the shoulders.

2. Stagger the legs apart, and create a kickstand by placing the top foot on the floor in front of the bottom foot; the heel of the top leg connects with the big toe of the bottom leg.

3. As you exhale, bracing the abs and lengthening the spine, push against the floor with the forearm and feet, lifting the side of the body off the floor; this is the side plank position. Keeping the body in a long, straight line, hold the position.

4. Curl the top arm downward and under the chest, turning the body in and under in the process.

5. As you inhale, uncurl the arm and body to return to the stacked side plank position.

6. Repeat the movement for repetitions or switch sides.

Regressions and Progressions

1. A regression is to bend the bottom knee and pull the bottom foot behind you to create a kickstand of support for the side plank.
2. A progression is to stack the top foot on top of the bottom foot for a greater stability challenge.

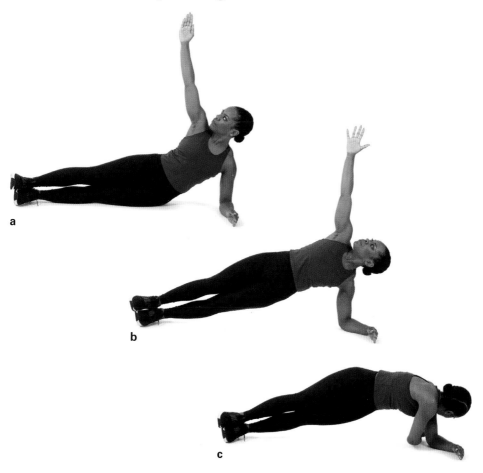

a

b

c

Safety Cues

1. Keep the abs engaged and active the entire time.
2. Find space between the ears and shoulders, not crunching in the neck. Think of long, straight spinal posture from the crown of the head all the way to the feet.

Variations

See the Regressions and Progressions section of this exercise for variations.

LEG RAISE

a

b

c

d

How It's Done

1. Start by lying in a supine position with the palms down, knees bent, and feet flat on the floor.
2. As you exhale, brace the abs, making them taut.
3. Rock the pelvis in and up, scooping the navel in and depressing the low back even more toward the floor.
4. As you inhale, lift both knees toward the chest and extend the legs straight up in the air; the heels are aligned over the hips.
5. Seal the thighs together, and stabilize the pelvis. The gaze is straight up.
6. As you exhale, hinge at the hips to lower the straight legs down toward the floor.
7. As you inhale, with a stronger bracing of the abs, lift the legs until the heels align over the hips.
8. Repeat for repetitions.

Regressions and Progressions

1. As a regression, some people find more support for their abs and back when they place the hands underneath the hips and butt during this exercise.
2. A progression is to lower the legs even lower, keeping the back on the floor, and hold at the bottom for a few seconds before lifting the legs back up.

Safety Cues

1. The low back should not lift up during this exercise. If it does, you have taken the legs too far down for your present range of motion.
2. Keep the head, back, and hips connected with the floor during this exercise.

Variations

1. Extend the arms overhead.
2. You may also add flutter kicks with the feet when the legs are lowered.

TOE TOUCH

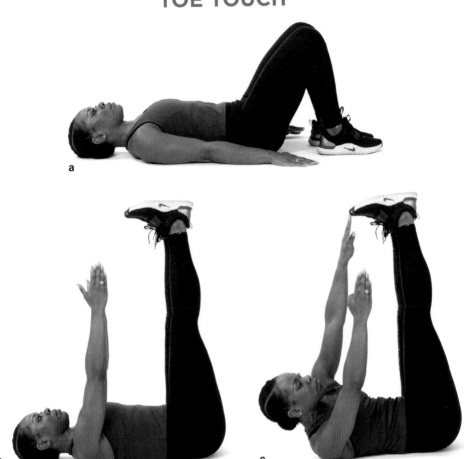

a

b

c

How It's Done

1. Start by lying in a supine position with the palms down, knees bent, and feet flat on the floor.
2. As you exhale, brace the abs, making them taut.
3. Rock the pelvis in and up, scooping the navel in and depressing the low back even more toward the floor.
4. As you inhale, lift both knees toward the chest and then extend the legs straight up in the air; the heels are aligned over the hips.
5. Seal the thighs together, and stabilize the pelvis. The gaze is straight up.
6. Lift the arms up until the wrists align with the shoulders.
7. As you exhale, lift the head, neck, and shoulders from the floor; you're in a crunch position.
8. Reach one hand and then the other for the toes; repeat for repetitions while alternating arm reaches.

Regressions and Progressions

1. Bending the knees is a regression.
2. A progression is to lift the shoulders higher off of the floor and reach past the feet each time you reach up.

Safety Cues

1. The low back and the back of the pelvis should remain on the floor.
2. If you experience tension in the neck or spine, rest from the exercise.

Variations

Perform this exercise with both feet on the floor and the knees bent, or with the knees bent at 90 degrees and the feet suspended to a supine tabletop or "dead bug" like position.

X SIT-UP

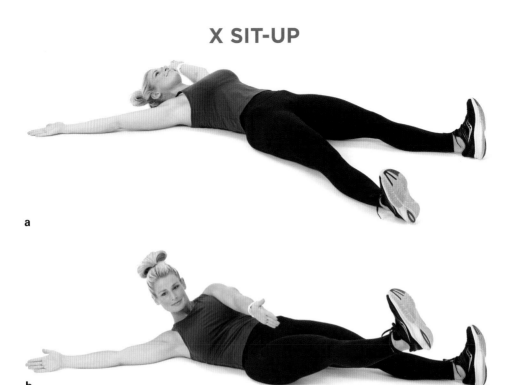

a

b

How It's Done

1. Start by lying in a supine position with the feet hip-width apart and the arms extended overhead and apart from each other. Your body should form the letter X.

2. Brace the abs, making them taut.

3. Rock the pelvis in and up, scooping the navel in and depressing the low back even more toward the floor.

4. As you exhale, lift one shoulder and the opposite leg from the floor. The arm will cross the midline of the body as you reach for the opposite ankle.

5. As you inhale, lower the limbs to the floor.

6. Repeat for repetitions, alternating sides with the other arm and leg.

ABS

Regressions and Progressions

1. A regression is to bend the knees more and not reach the arms as high.
2. A progression is to reach higher and longer with the arms and legs for a deeper abdominal crunch.

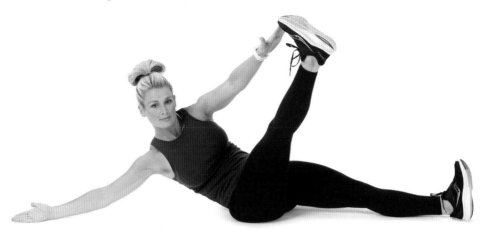

Safety Cues

1. The pelvis should remain stabilized and neutral throughout this exercise. The hips should not lift from the floor.
2. Keep bracing the abs for better spinal stabilization and abdominal work.

Variations

See the Regressions and Progressions section of this exercise for variations.

CHAPTER 7

Warm-Up and Activation Exercises

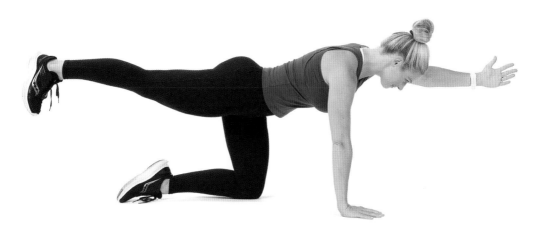

Before exercising the core, it's helpful to first turn on and prime the abs and glutes so that you can achieve maximal activation during the strengthening phase. Because most adults in the United States spend a great majority of their time seated for extended periods (e.g., in the car, at a work desk, during meals), the glutes are often dormant and deactivated. In addition, poor posture accounts for weak abs. Prolonged sitting and poor posture have a negative effect on muscle activation, tone, and strength.

Wake up your muscles by starting every workout with mobility and muscular activation moves that mimic the focused muscle movement patterns of the workout. Properly warming up the body prepares the joints and muscles of the kinetic chain to perform well for maximal exercise results.

The following warm-up and activation sequence can be performed using body weight, but light resistance bands are optional. Bands can be used as a great tool to help control range of motion and focus on optimal form. This sequence should take 5 to 7 minutes; for each move, perform 10 to 12 repetitions (reps).

STANDING LEG SWING

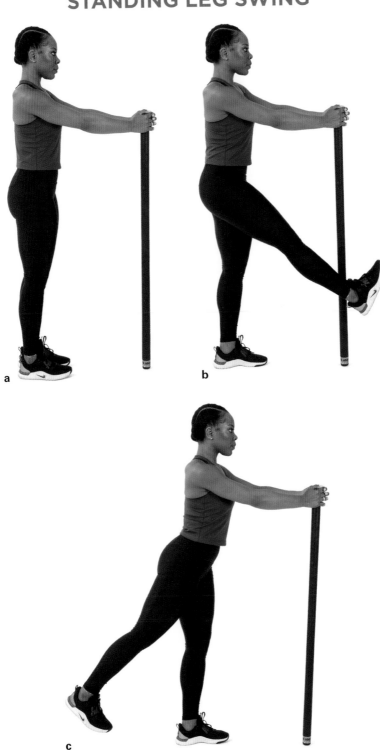

How It's Done

1. Stand tall with the chest lifted and proud, torso long, shoulders stacked over hips, hips over knees, and knees over heels. Grip the top of a weighted bar or barbell with both hands. Look directly forward.
2. Softly bend both knees for balance support.
3. Keeping the hips squared forward, lift one foot up slightly. Swing the leg forward and back from the hip socket while maintaining a firm grip on the bar.
4. Lower the foot to the starting position, and repeat the exercise on the other side.

Regressions and Progressions

1. Hold on to a stable surface for additional balance support.
2. Depending on your level of flexibility and balance, swing your leg higher and farther.

Safety and Form

1. Stay balanced, and keep the shoulders and hips squared in the same direction.
2. Keep the torso tall and abs strong.

CORE ACTIVATION

STANDING HURDLER

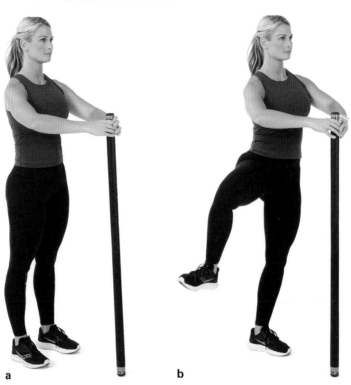

a   b

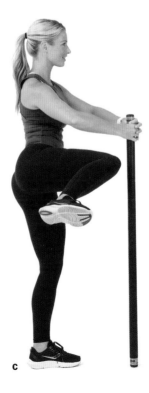

c

How It's Done

1. Stand tall with the chest lifted and proud, torso long, shoulders stacked over hips, hips over knees, and knees over heels. Grip the top of a weighted bar or barbell with both hands. Look directly forward.
2. Pick up one foot, opening the hip. Lift the knee up to the side, then pull the knee around to the front, closing the hip.
3. Land the foot back down to the starting position.
4. Repeat the exercise on the other side. Alternate sides for reps.

Regressions and Progressions

1. Hold on to a stable surface for additional balance support.
2. Make this move athletic by moving forward and back rather than standing in place.

Safety and Form

1. Stabilize the pelvis, and keep the abs strong.
2. Allow the arms to move naturally as they would if you were walking.

CORE ACTIVATION

REVERSE LUNGE WITH SIDE REACH

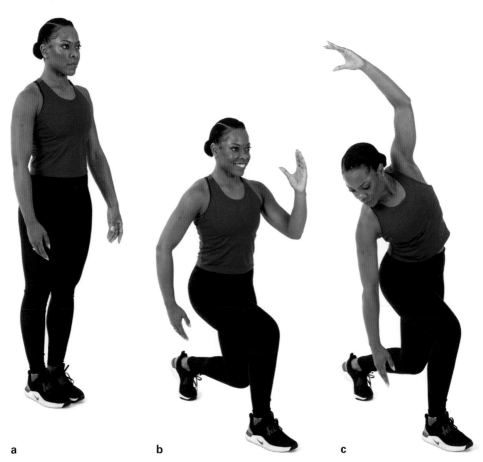

a   b   c

How It's Done

1. Stand tall with the chest lifted and proud, torso long, shoulders stacked over hips, hips over knees, and knees over heels. Look directly forward.
2. Step one foot far back behind you, bending both knees at a 90-degree angle.
3. Bending the knees, lower straight down, keeping the chest up.
4. Hover the back knee over the floor, and reach the arm opposite of the front knee up and over for a side-body stretch. You will feel a lengthening sensation in your side and hip flexor.
5. Step in, return to the starting position, and repeat the movement on the other side.

Regressions and Progressions

1. A regression is to shorten your range of motion or eliminate the side stretch.
2. A progression is to reach your arm farther over or lower deeper into the lunge.

Safety and Form

1. Be sure to step far enough back so that the front knee does not pass the front toes.
2. Keep the torso tall, shoulders back, and chest lifted and proud while performing this move.

CORE ACTIVATION

LATERAL LUNGE WITH SIDE LEG LIFT

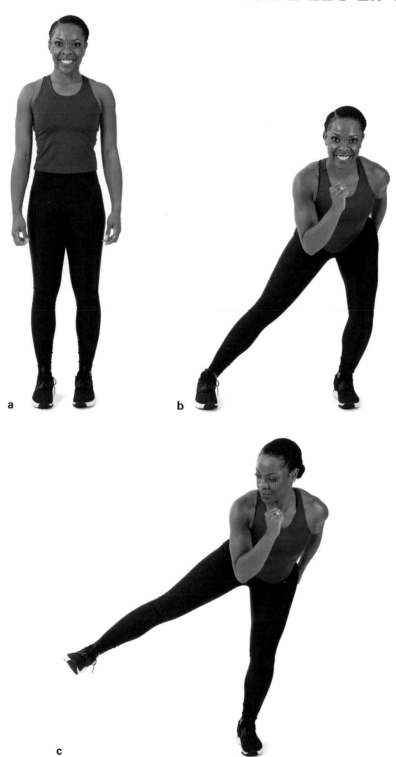

a

b

c

How It's Done

1. Stand tall with the chest lifted and proud, torso long, shoulders stacked over hips, hips over knees, and knees over heels. Look directly forward.
2. Take a wide step to the side (for this example, start with the left foot), bending the left knee toward 90 degrees as the foot lands. The toes and knees are pointing in the same direction.
3. Lift the right leg up and out to the side, keeping the leg extended, engaging the glutes and abs.
4. Land the right foot, and step the left foot back in toward the right foot, returning to the starting position.
5. Repeat the movement on the other side, starting with the right leg.

Regressions and Progressions

1. Omit the side leg lift for a regression.
2. Deepen the side lunge for added muscular challenge.

Safety and Form

1. Be sure that all 10 toes and both knees point forward as you step to the side and lunge.
2. Bracing the abs and activating the glutes before moving is ideal for balance and stability.

CORE ACTIVATION

DOWNWARD-FACING DOG TO PLANK

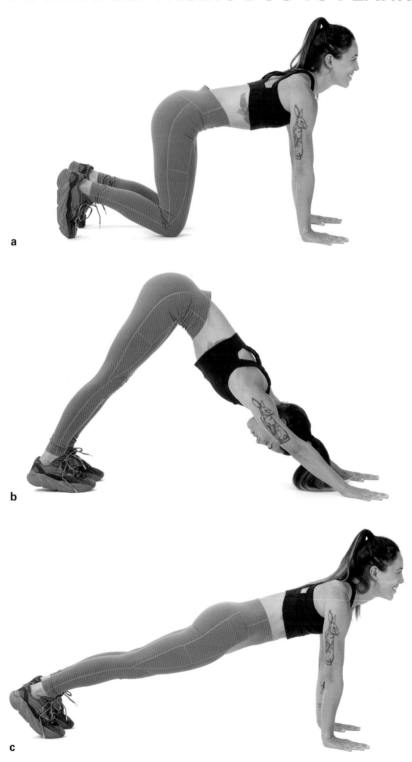

a

b

c

How It's Done

1. Begin on all fours in a tabletop position, aligning the hands directly under the shoulders and the knees under the hips.
2. As you exhale, press the palms and toes firmly into the floor, lift the knees, extend the legs, and press the hips back until you are in an inverted position (downward-facing dog).
3. As you inhale, shift your body forward until it is straight and parallel to the floor in a plank position. The hands are directly under the shoulders, and the abs are engaged.
4. Repeat the sequence, pushing the palms and toes firmly into the floor and lifting back into downward-facing dog.

Regressions and Progressions

1. Keep a bend in the knees as needed depending on leg flexibility.
2. Tabletop to child's pose is a regressive option.
3. As a progression, lift one leg at a time in downward-facing dog and plank.

Safety and Form

1. In downward-facing dog, the ears are in between the biceps, the hips stay lifted, and the heels of the feet are pressing toward the floor.
2. You should not have to move your hands and feet when moving between downward-facing dog and plank.
3. Keep the spine long and abs engaged, and keep breathing deeply the entire time.

CORE ACTIVATION

BIRDDOG WITH LATERAL ARM AND LEG REACH

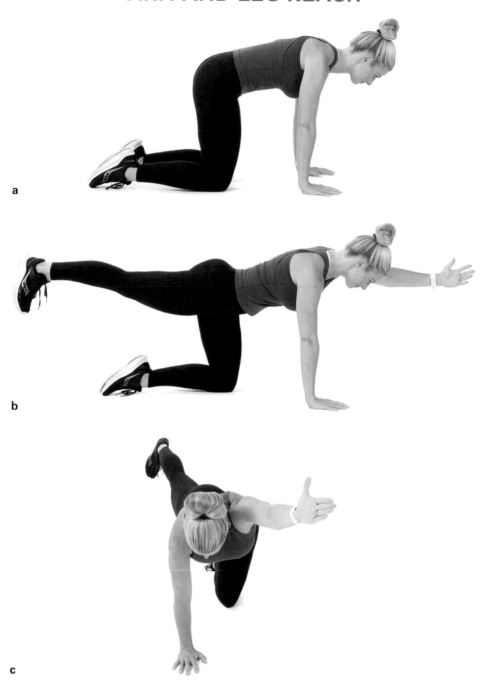

a

b

c

How It's Done

1. Begin on all fours, aligning the hands directly under the shoulders and the knees under the hips.
2. Extend the left arm and right leg simultaneously until both limbs are parallel to the floor.
3. Dorsiflex the right ankle so that the right toes point down toward the floor. The left shoulder and right hip should be aligned with the torso.
4. Once the left arm and right leg are fully extended and you are balancing on the right palm and left knee, exhale, taking the left arm and right leg out to an angle.
5. Return the left arm and right leg back to center; balance, then lower the limbs to the floor, returning to the starting position on all fours.
6. Repeat steps 2 through 5 with the right arm and left leg.

Regressions and Progressions

1. For a regression option to help with balance, extend a single arm and return it to the floor first, then extend a single opposite leg and return it.
2. For more of a challenge, hold the extended arm and leg on the diagonal for 10 seconds before returning to your starting position.

Safety and Form

1. Keep the spine long and abs braced the entire time.
2. The shoulders and hips should remain aligned with the torso.
3. Put something soft under the knees for extra cushion.

CORE ACTIVATION

COBRA

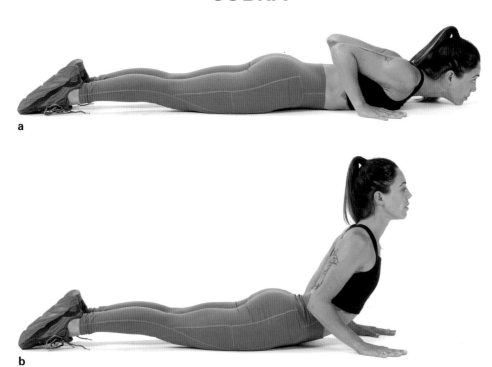

a

b

How It's Done

1. Start in a prone position (lying flat on the abdomen) with the legs extended behind you. The palms are under the shoulders and pressing into the floor.
2. Engaging the glutes and back muscles as you exhale, press into the floor with the palms, lifting the chest forward and upward. You will feel a stretch along the front of your body.
3. Disengage the glutes and back muscles as you slowly lower to the starting position.

Regressions and Progressions

1. A regression is to lessen your range of motion upon lifting away from the floor.
2. A progression is to push your palms deeper into the floor as you lift the front of your body completely from the floor, stabilizing on the palms and the tops of the feet in upward-facing dog.

Safety and Form

1. Depress the shoulders away from the ears.
2. Lift the chest forward and upward to avoid compressing or pinching in the low back.

CORE ACTIVATION

SUPINE PELVIC TILT TO BENT-KNEE LIFT

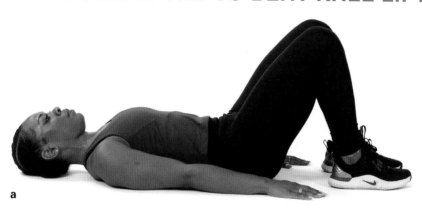

a

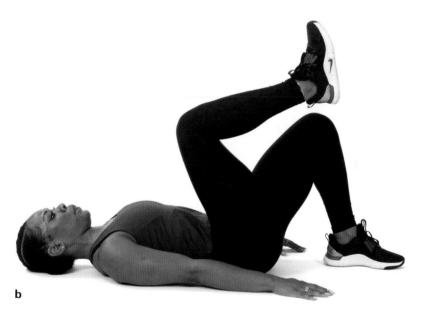

b

How It's Done

1. Start by lying in a supine position with the palms down, knees bent, and feet flat on the floor.

2. As you exhale, brace the abs, making them taut. The muscles you are focusing on are the pelvic floor muscles that engage when you let out a big laugh or cough.

3. Rock the pelvis in and up, scooping the navel in and depressing the low back even more toward the floor.

4. Keeping this engagement in the abs, lift one knee toward the chest, then lower it back down; lift the other knee toward the chest, then lower it back down.

5. With both feet flat on the floor, release the abdominal bracing, rock the pelvis away from the stomach, and return to the starting position.

Regressions and Progressions

1. You can perform the pelvic tilt with abdominal bracing without lifting the knees.

2. For more abdominal challenge, lift both knees simultaneously.

Safety and Form

The goal is to keep the entire back and hips relatively connected with the floor. Of course, be mindful of the natural curvature of your own spine.

CORE ACTIVATION

GLUTE BRIDGE WITH ABDUCTION

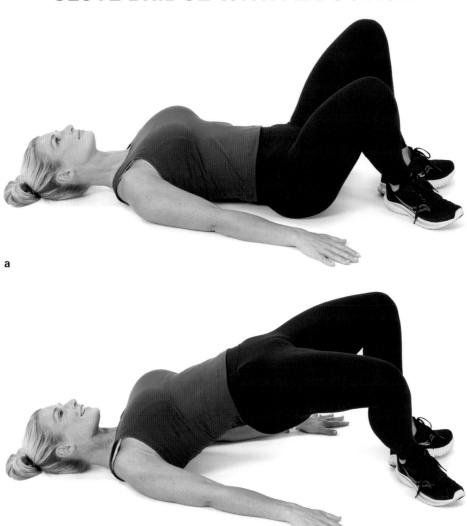

a

b

How It's Done

1. Start by lying in a supine position with the palms down, knees comfortably bent, and feet flat on the floor in a turned-out position with heels together. The feet and thighs make a V shape.
2. Press the feet firmly into the floor, activate the glutes, and lift the hips up. The spine should form a long line.
3. Balancing on the backs of the shoulders, control the movement as you continue to open the knees apart in a V position. You should feel the tops and outer edges of the glutes engaged.
4. With control, slowly close the knees back to the starting point, disengage the glutes, and lower the hips to the starting position.

Regressions and Progressions

1. Shortening your range of motion is an optional regression.
2. Loop a resistance band around the thighs (above the knees) for more gluteal activation.

Safety and Form

1. You should not feel aches or pains in the knees. If you do, step both feet away from the glutes to add distance between the heels and butt.
2. You should not lift your hips so high that you feel tightness in the low back. If you feel pain in the low back as you lift the hips, perhaps you have lifted too high.
3. If using a resistance band, keep tension in the band the entire time.

CORE ACTIVATION

SIDE-LYING CLAM

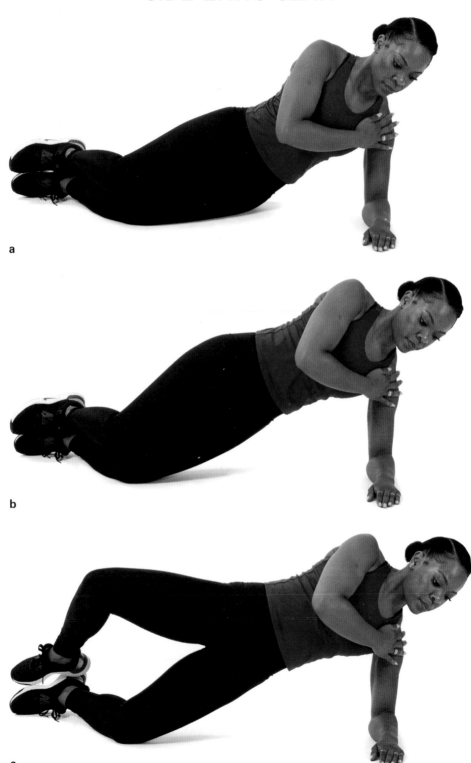

a

b

c

How It's Done

1. Start in a side-lying position with the bottom forearm on the floor and the elbow under the shoulder. The legs are stacked, the feet are pulled behind you, and the knees are bent toward a 90-degree angle.
2. Place the top hand across the chest onto the opposite shoulder to stabilize the torso.
3. Lift the hips up into a side plank position, and hold that position.
4. Keeping the bottom knee on the floor, lift the top knee up, opening the knees apart. You should feel the tops and outer edges of the glutes engaged.
5. Close the top knee down, then slowly lower both hips back to the floor.

Regressions and Progressions

1. A regression is to keep the hips and side of the body on the floor with the bottom arm extended, head relaxed on that arm, and knees in front of the hips instead of lifting up into a side plank.
2. Loop a resistance band around the thighs (above the knees) for more gluteal activation. Keep tension in the band the entire time.

Safety and Form

1. Be sure that the hip bones are stacked on top of one another.
2. Brace the abs to stabilize the pelvis and torso during this movement.

CORE ACTIVATION

LUNGING HIP THRUSTER

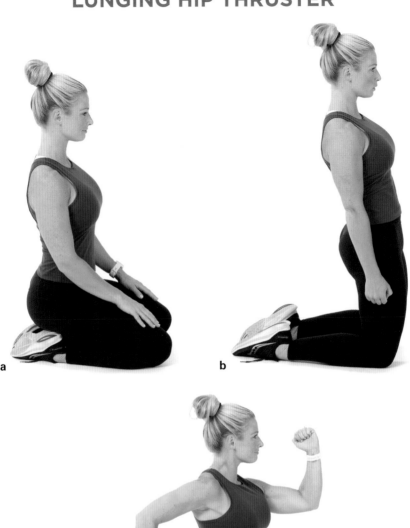

a

b

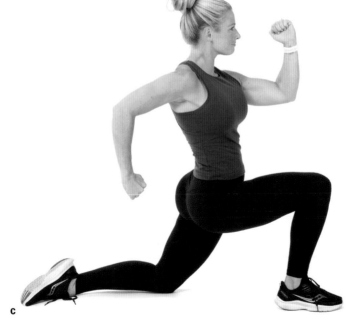

c

How It's Done

1. Start in a kneeling position on the floor, sitting on the heels.
2. Brace the abs and activate the glutes as you lift the butt away from the heels, driving the hips forward. You are standing on the knees with the thighs and torso forming an upright, straight line.
3. Step forward with the right foot while still driving the hips forward. The left arm moves forward, and the right arm moves back in a runner's stance.
4. Disengage the glutes as you slowly move the right foot back and lower the hips to sit on the heels.
5. Repeat the movement with the left leg stepping forward.

Regressions and Progressions

1. Place a soft cushion under the knees for support.
2. For added gluteal activation, anchor a resistance band to a grounded object behind you that will not move. Step inside the looped band, and place the band low around the hips; you are facing away from the anchor point. Keep the band taut as you perform the move.

Safety and Form

1. Keep the shoulders, hips, knees, and ankles squared.
2. Keep the torso tall and long while performing this move.

CORE ACTIVATION

STANDING TAP-OUT AND TAPBACK

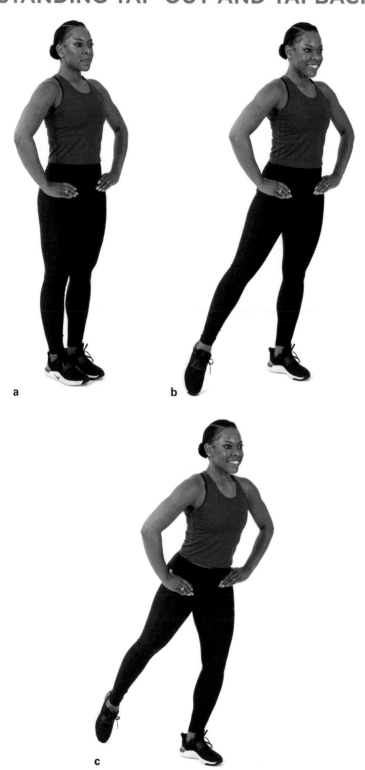

a

b

c

How It's Done

1. Stand tall with the chest lifted and proud, torso long, shoulders stacked over hips, hips over knees, and knees over heels. The feet are slightly wider than hip-distance apart. Place the hands squarely on the hips, and look directly forward.

2. Step the right foot out to the side without moving the left leg or pelvis out of alignment and without transferring your weight from the stabilizing leg. Return the foot to the starting position.

3. Keeping the torso, pelvis, and left leg stable, tap the right big toe back, and do not land the heel. Return the foot to the starting position.

4. Repeat the movement with the left leg.

Regressions and Progressions

1. Shorten your range of motion for a regression.

2. Add a resistance band around both legs (just above the ankles) for added gluteal activation. Keep the band taut as you perform the move.

Safety and Form

1. Keep the abs braced and the body tall while performing this move.

2. Breathe deeply while performing this move.

3. Keep a soft bend in the knees, and keep the shoulders and hands relaxed.

CORE ACTIVATION

CHAPTER 8
Stretches

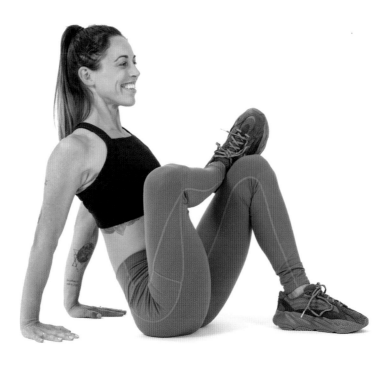

Stretching after your workout is beneficial for muscle recovery, reducing muscle tension and soreness, injury prevention, improved range of motion, and preparing the mind and body for the next workout to come. The cool-down and stretch are just as important as the warm-up and workout; they should never be negated.

The following recovery moves are performed with only your body weight. The focus of these stretches is to find length in the muscles used primarily during the ab and glute workouts. Hold each stretch for about 10 seconds. You have the option to hold the stretches longer or repeat stretches if it feels good to your body. This sequence should take about 5 to 7 minutes.

You are encouraged to take whatever stretch your body needs to release tightness and help alleviate muscle soreness.

HIP FLEXOR STRETCH

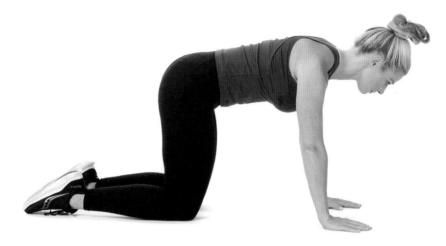

a

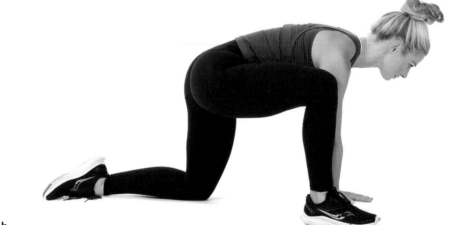

b

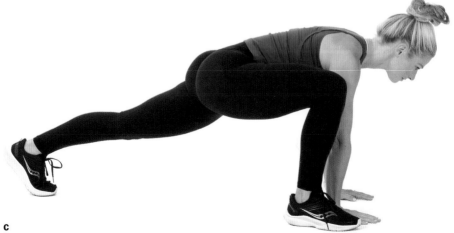

c

How It's Done

1. Start on all fours in a tabletop position, aligning the hands directly under the shoulders and the knees under the hips. The spine is neutral and long.
2. Step one foot forward to the side of the palms.
3. Rock the shoulders up, back, and down to help keep the upper body stable in a neutral position.
4. Send the hips forward, keeping the front knee stacked over the ankle. You will feel a stretch in the upper thigh and hip of the back leg.
5. Step the foot back, returning the body to tabletop position, then switch sides.

Regressions and Progressions

1. To lessen the intensity of the stretch for a regression, try not stepping the foot as far forward or sending the hips as far forward.
2. To increase your range of motion for a progression, step the foot farther forward, and place the palms on the thigh or extend the arms overhead as you send the hips forward.

Safety Cues

1. Ensure the knee remains stacked over the ankle.
2. Keep the spine neutral and long; avoid rounding in the spine.

STANDING BACKBEND

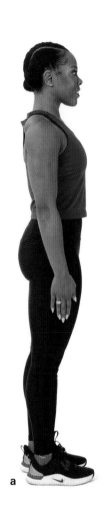

a

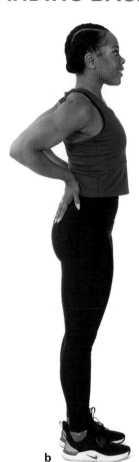

b

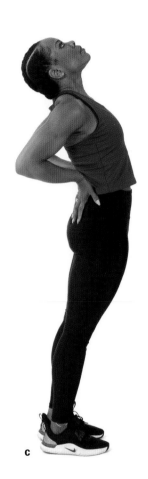

c

How It's Done

1. Stand tall with the chest lifted and proud, torso long, shoulders stacked over hips, hips over knees, and knees over heels. Relax the arms at the sides, and look directly forward.
2. Place the palms on the small of the back with the fingers pointing down toward the backs of the heels.
3. Circle the shoulders back and down.
4. As you exhale, activate the glutes, drive the pelvis forward, arch the back, and gaze up. You should feel the stretch along the front of your body.
5. As you inhale, disengage the glutes, returning to standing.

Regressions and Progressions

1. Shorten your range of motion for a regression.
2. Extend the lever by reaching the arms up and overhead while you stretch back to intensify the stretch along the front of your body.

Safety Cues

1. Keep your weight distributed in between all four corners of the feet, and keep the knees softly bent.
2. Move with your breath to discourage dizziness.

STANDING LATERAL EXTENSION

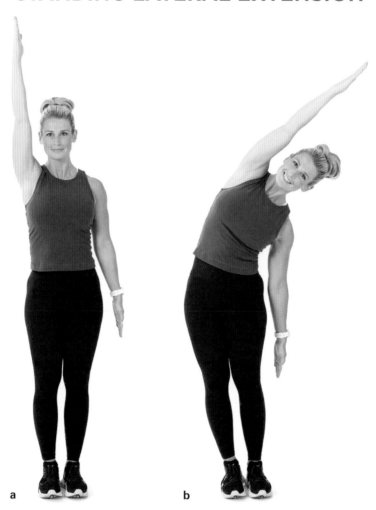

a   b

How It's Done

1. Stand tall with the shoulders back and down, chest lifted and proud, torso long, shoulders stacked over hips, hips over knees, and knees over heels. Relax the arms at the sides, and look directly forward.

2. Lift one arm overhead (for this example, start with the right arm); keep the left arm down at the side.

3. Push the right hip to the side, slightly bending the left knee, and reach the right arm up and over the midline of your body. You should feel the length and stretch along the right side of your body.

4. Brace the abs, and return to standing. Release the right arm to the side.

5. Repeat the stretch with the left arm.

Regressions and Progressions

1. Shorten your lever by bending in the extended arm and placing the palm behind your head to help alleviate the intensity of the stretch.

2. Crossed-leg lateral extension is a progression of the stretch. For example, cross the right leg over the left with the right foot placed solidly on the ground as you reach the right arm up and over to intensify the side-body stretch.

Safety Cues

1. You may hold on to a wall or stable surface to help keep your balance.

2. You may bend the knees more to help with stability, balance, and range of motion in this stretch.

STRETCHES FOR THE CORE

COW POSE

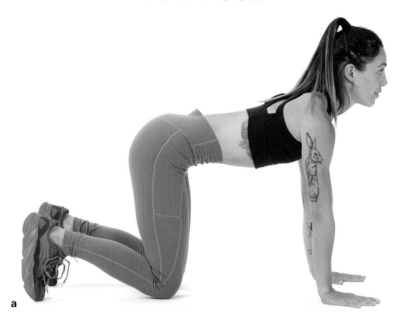

a

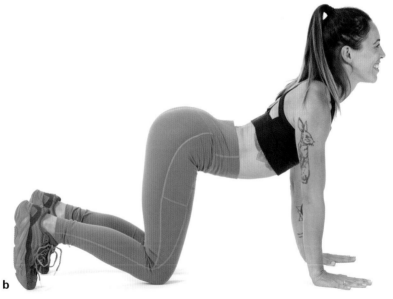

b

How It's Done

1. Start on all fours in a tabletop position, aligning the hands directly under the shoulders and the knees under the hips. The spine is long from the crown of the head to the tailbone. The gaze is straight ahead (as in the photo), or it is recommended to be down at the space between both palms.
2. As you inhale, reach the crown of the head forward and the tailbone back to make space between the vertebrae.
3. Scoop the crown of the head and tailbone upward as you gaze forward and upward.
4. As you exhale, return to tabletop position.

Regressions and Progressions

1. For a regression, see the cobra exercise in chapter 7.
2. For a progression, try upward-facing dog (see the progression for cobra in chapter 7).

Safety Cues

1. Remember to keep your spine long and your shoulders relaxed from your ears.
2. The goal is to find space between each vertebra, not to crunch in your back. Think length and stretch.

STRETCHES FOR THE CORE

TABLETOP TAIL WAG

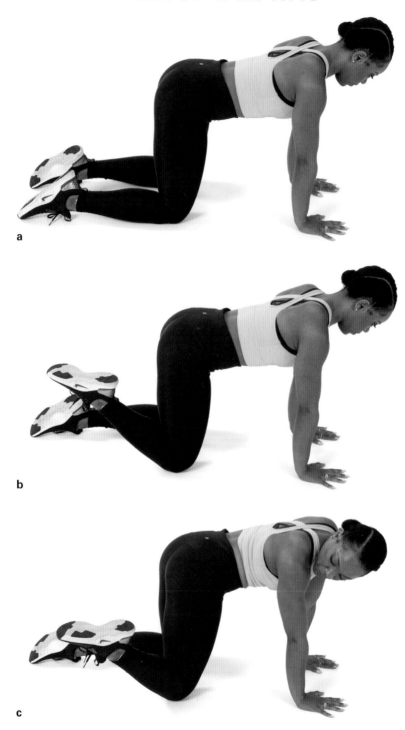

a

b

c

How It's Done

1. Start on all fours in a tabletop position, aligning the hands directly under the shoulders and the knees under the hips. The spine is long from the crown of the head to the tailbone. The gaze is toward the floor, at the space between both palms.
2. Lift one foot (for this example, start with the right foot) while keeping the right knee on the floor.
3. Sweep the right foot out to the right side while crunching along the right side of your body to look back at the right foot. You will feel a stretch on the left side of the torso.
4. Release the side-body crunch, and return to the starting position.
5. Repeat the stretch on the left side.

Regressions and Progressions

1. Add a cushion under the knees for comfort.
2. Lateral child's pose is a progression. Press the hips back to the heels while reaching both arms over to one side and then the other.

Safety Cues

1. Remember to keep the spine long, with the shoulders relaxed and away from the ears.
2. The goal is to find space between each vertebra, not to crunch the spine. Think of length and stretch for one side of your body at a time.

SUPINE TWIST

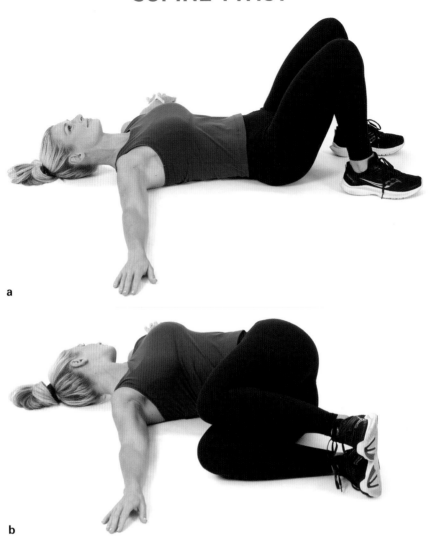

a

b

How It's Done

1. Lie supine with the knees comfortably bent and the feet flat on the floor.
2. Open both arms out wide to make a letter T. Keep the backs of the shoulders connected to the floor.
3. Connect the thighs. With control, drop both knees over to one side as you turn your head to look the opposite way. You will feel a twist and stretch in the torso and hips.
4. Brace the abs to lift the knees and return to the starting position.
5. Repeat the twist in the opposite direction.

Regressions and Progressions

1. Keep your gaze up and don't turn your head while you twist for a regression.
2. Another regression is to decrease your range of motion by not dropping your knees as far over to the side.
3. Lift the knees to stack over the hips before dropping them over to one side in the twist for a progression.

Safety Cues

Pay attention to how the back responds to this stretch. If you experience pain or excessive tightness in the back, do not do this stretch.

QUADRICEPS STRETCH

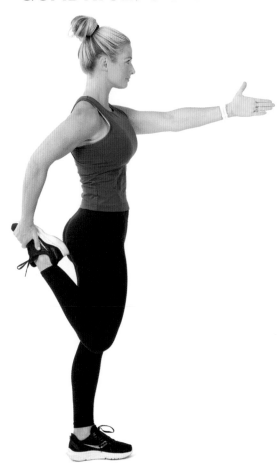

How It's Done

1. Start by standing tall with the shoulders back and down, chest and spine neutral, and hips stacked over the feet.
2. Shift your weight over to one side to balance on that same leg.
3. Kick the opposite heel toward the butt, and catch the front of that foot in the same-side hand.
4. Close the knee toward the midline of your body.
5. Continue to pull the heel toward the butt to feel the stretch in the quadriceps.
6. Release the hand from the foot, and place the foot on the floor to return to the starting position.
7. Perform the stretch on the other side.

Regressions and Progressions

1. Wrap a towel or strap around the ankle, and grip it to assist your reach to the foot.
2. To decrease or increase the intensity of the stretch, vary the range of motion of how far you take the heel toward the butt and how tall you stand.

Safety Cues

If balance is a challenge for you, hold on to a wall or other stable surface to help keep your balance.

SEATED FIGURE 4

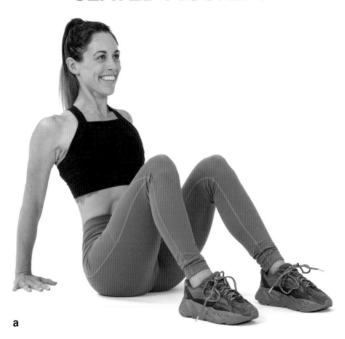

a

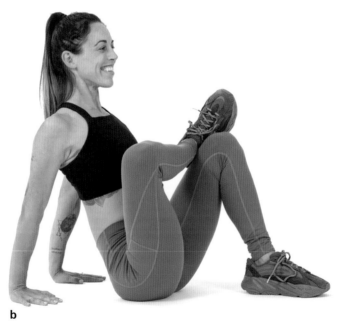

b

How It's Done

1. Start in a seated position with the knees bent and the feet flat on the floor. The palms are on the floor to the sides and slightly behind you with the fingertips pointing forward.
2. Place one ankle across the other knee (for this example, right ankle over left knee); the right knee points out to the right.
3. Walk the hands forward, closer to the body, to prop yourself up and sit taller. You will feel the stretch in the right hip and glutes.
4. Release the stretch, and repeat it on the left side.

Regressions and Progressions

1. Try a supine figure 4 for less intensity on the lower back as a regression. Lying supine, cross one ankle over the opposite knee, then hug the knees in toward the chest.
2. Try a pigeon pose for a progression. Pigeon pose increases the range of motion at the hip for a deeper hip and glute stretch. From all fours, move one leg forward, bringing the knee toward the same-side wrist and the ankle toward the opposite-side wrist. Slide the other leg back to extend it long.

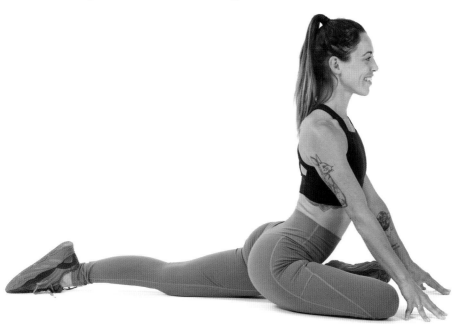

Safety Cues

Accept your own level of flexibility, and do not force the stretch. Stop before you feel pain.

HAMSTRING STRETCH

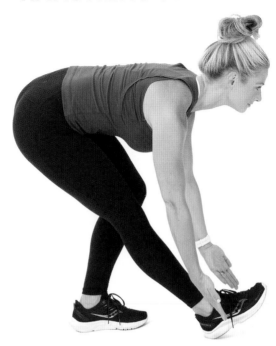

How It's Done

1. Stand tall with the chest up and proud, torso long, shoulders stacked over hips, hips over knees, and knees over heels. Relax the arms at the sides, and look directly forward.
2. Extend one heel out in front of you like a kickstand, and dig it into the ground. Keep the leg extended long.
3. Bend the knee of the stabilizing leg, send the hips back, the arms forward, and bow the torso forward. You will feel the stretch in the back of the right leg.
4. Return to standing and switch sides.

Regressions and Progressions

1. Stay more upright for less stretch.
2. Hold this stretch for a few deep breaths; each time you exhale move deeper into the stretch.

Safety Cues

1. Keep a bend in the stabilizing knee for balance and for greater range of motion in the stretch.
2. Keep the spine long, shoulders back and down, and chest expansive during the stretch.

HAPPY BABY

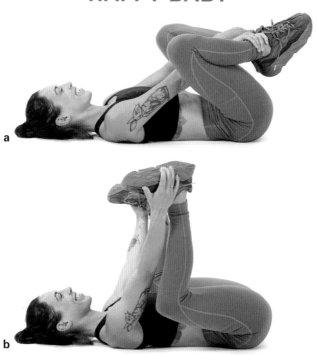

a

b

How It's Done

1. Lie supine with the head relaxed to the floor, the knees pulled into the chest, and the hips turned out so that the knees are opened wide.
2. Reach the palms forward, and grab the outside edges of the feet. Lift the feet up toward the sky, bending the knees and pressing them down and out toward the sides of your body.
3. Gently pull down on the feet, depressing the hips to the floor. You will feel an opening sensation in the inner thighs, hips, and groin.

Regressions and Progressions

1. If you are unable to reach the flexed feet, try holding on to the back of your bent knees and pull down gently.
2. For a progression, extend the legs long while holding on to the blade edges of your feet.

Safety Cues

1. Keep the head, neck, and shoulders relaxed to the floor to avoid unnecessary tension on the spine.
2. Flex the feet and pull the knees down and in toward the outer sides of the chest, pressing the back of the hips down toward the floor.

BUTTERFLY

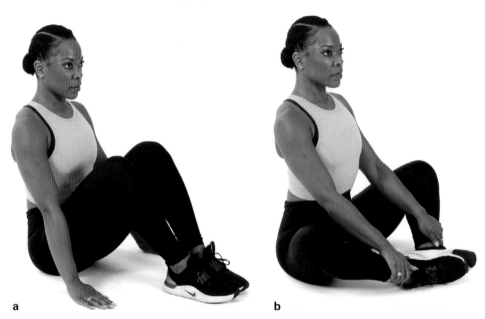

a

b

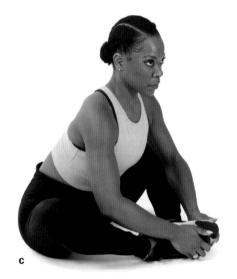

c

How It's Done

1. Start in a seated position with the knees bent and both feet flat on the floor.
2. Open both knees outward, and bring the soles of the feet together.
3. Inhale; as you exhale, bow the chest forward while keeping the sit bones connected with the floor. You will feel the stretch in the groin, hips, and top of your butt.

Regressions and Progressions

1. Shortening your range of motion when opening your knees is an optional regression. You can also omit the fold or bow forward to lessen the intensity.
2. A progression is to gently add pressure by placing the palms on the inner thighs and pressing to open the knees wider.

Safety Cues

1. Be sure the sit bones remain connected with the floor.
2. Keep the spine long when folding forward.

STRETCHES FOR THE CORE

SEATED WINDSHIELD WIPER

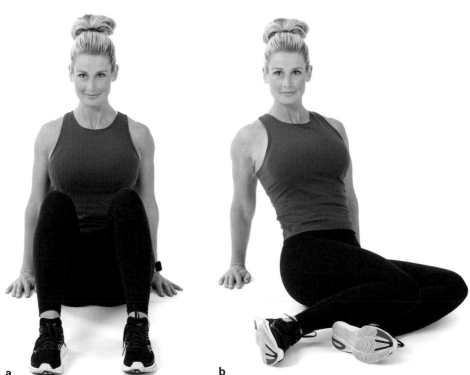

a   b

How It's Done

1. Start in an upright seated position with the knees bent and the soles of the feet flat on the floor. The palms are on the floor with the fingertips pointing forward, just to the sides of the hips. The feet are hip-width apart.
2. Drop both knees to one side, making a sweeping motion like a windshield wiper. You will feel the hips stretch and release tension.
3. Return the knees and feet to the starting position, and sweep them to the other side.

Regressions and Progressions

1. Shortening your range of motion when dropping the knees over to the side is an optional regression.
2. A progression is to twist the torso in opposition to the knees as they drop to one side.

Safety Cues

1. Keep the torso upright and tall throughout this movement.
2. If you experience tightness or tension in the bent knees, step the heels farther away from your hips.

PART IV

CORE WORKOUTS

CHAPTER 9

Core Endurance-Focused Workouts

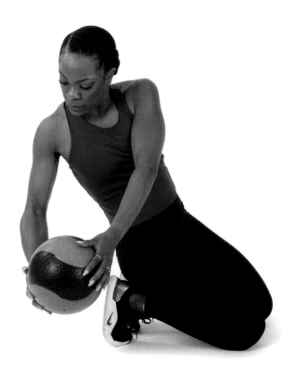

Muscular endurance is the ability of a muscle to repeatedly exert force, perform multiple repetitions of an exercise, and remain active over an extended period. Think of it as running a marathon rather than a sprint. Typically, endurance-focused training is performed with less resistance, less weight, or body-weight only in order to sustain the exercises for a longer period before muscular fatigue or failure. The goal is to perform quality movement patterns for higher repetitions. Compromise of form is a sign to end the exercise set and rest before continuing to the next set.

The workouts in this chapter combine exercises performed front to back, side to side, and in rotation. These exercises are presented and explained in part III of this book. Revisit part III for exercise descriptions and cueing; page numbers for the exercises are included with the workouts. You can plug in and play with any of the core exercises presented in this book to create a personal core endurance-focused workout; you do not have to stick to only what is presented in this section.

You are strongly encouraged to effectively warm up with the dynamic warm-up program found in chapter 7 before doing any of these workouts. Properly warming up will prepare the body for optimal performance and maximal exercise results. The warm-up is not accounted for in the workout period you see for each workout; your warm-up should take you between 5 and 7 minutes to complete. Also not accounted for is the time you spend cooling down and stretching with stretches found in chapter 8, which should also take between 5 and 7 minutes. The suggested times for your workouts are based on the performance of the average adult exerciser in the United States. The time, sets, repetitions (reps), resistances, and rest periods presented in these workouts are merely suggestions; adjust them to suit your evolving fitness level and ability. You may also choose to do only one or two of the sequences from either of the full workouts in this chapter at the end of a cardio-focused workout (before the cool-down) to add some strength work to your workout.

Workout 1: Abs With Focus on Muscular Endurance

Workout period: 20 to 30 minutes

Number of exercises per workout sequence: 4 or 5 exercises

Sets: 2 or 3 sets for each exercise; rest periods of 30 seconds or less between each set of each exercise

Reps: At least 12 reps per set or per your personal preference

Resistance: Body weight or your definition of lighter resistance bands or weights; in other words, weight under 65 percent of your one-repetition maximum (1RM; the maximum weight you can lift for only one repetition with optimal and proper form and alignment)

SAMPLE ENDURANCE-FOCUSED AB WORKOUT

WORKOUT SEQUENCE 1: COMBO AB EXERCISES		
Exercise	**Exercise photo**	**Page number**
1. Forward flexion to knee		60
2. K-crunch		110
3. Bicycle		120
4. Sumo lateral crunch		68

(continued)

Sample Endurance-Focused Ab Workout *(continued)*

WORKOUT SEQUENCE 1: COMBO AB EXERCISES *(continued)*		
Exercise	**Exercise photo**	**Page number**
5. Thread the needle		130
WORKOUT SEQUENCE 2: FLOOR AB EXERCISES A		
Exercise	**Exercise photo**	**Page number**
1. Pilates roll-up		116
2. Side plank		122
3. Windshield wiper		124
4. Leg raise		132
5. X sit-up		136

WORKOUT SEQUENCE 3: STANDING-ONLY AB EXERCISES		
Exercise	**Exercise photo**	**Page number**
1. Anterior pelvic tilt		72
2. Lateral flexion to knee		62
3. Sumo crossbody reach		64
4. Side hip tuck		74
5. Crossbody knee drive		66

(continued)

Sample Endurance-Focused Ab Workout *(continued)*

WORKOUT SEQUENCE 4: FLOOR AB EXERCISES B		
Exercise	**Exercise photo**	**Page number**
1. Abdominal pushout		114
2. Side crunch		106
3. Kneeling torso twist		112
4. V-sit		108

Workout 2: Glutes With Focus on Muscular Endurance

Workout period: 20 to 30 minutes

Number of exercises per workout sequence: 4 or 5 exercises

Sets: 2 or 3 sets for each exercise; rest periods of 30 seconds or less between each set of each exercise

Reps: At least 12 reps per set or per your personal preference

Resistance: Body weight or your definition of lighter resistance bands or weights; in other words, weight under 65 percent of your one-repetition maximum (1RM; the maximum weight you can lift for only one repetition with optimal and proper form and alignment)

SAMPLE ENDURANCE-FOCUSED GLUTE WORKOUT

WORKOUT SEQUENCE 1: COMBO GLUTE EXERCISES		
Exercise	Exercise photo	Page number
1. Squat		40
2. Lunge		44
3. Sumo squat		50
4. Fire hydrant		88

(continued)

Sample Endurance-Focused Glute Workout *(continued)*

WORKOUT SEQUENCE 1: COMBO GLUTE EXERCISES *(continued)*		
Exercise	**Exercise photo**	**Page number**
5. Bridge with knee abduction		86

WORKOUT SEQUENCE 2: FLOOR-ONLY GLUTE EXERCISES		
Exercise	**Exercise photo**	**Page number**
1. Single-leg bridge		90
2. Donkey kick		94
3. Frogger		96
4. Clam		100
5. Seal heel clap		102

WORKOUT SEQUENCE 3: STANDING-ONLY GLUTE EXERCISES		
Exercise	**Exercise photo**	**Page number**
1. Squat to standing leg raise		40, 56
2. Standing tap-out and tapback		162
3. Sumo squat to lateral lunge		50,52
4. Squat tapback		42
5. Pistol squat		54

(continued)

Sample Endurance-Focused Glute Workout *(continued)*

WORKOUT SEQUENCE 4: COMBO GLUTE AND AB EXERCISES		
Exercise	**Exercise photo**	**Page number**
1. Sumo squat to lateral flexion to knee		50, 62
2. Lateral lunge to cross-body knee drive		52, 66
3. Decline hip bridge to windshield wiper		80, 124
4. Extended reverse leg lift to plank saw		98, 126

CHAPTER 10

Glute Hypertrophy-Focused Workouts

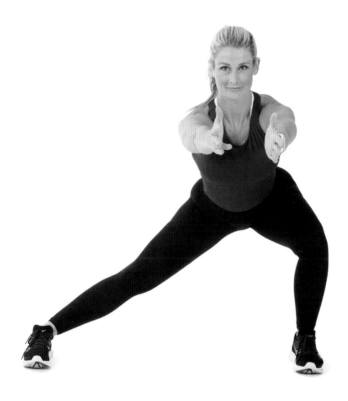

Muscular hypertrophy is the enlargement of muscle mass. It is more common in fast-twitch muscle fibers than in slow-twitch muscle fibers. With hypertrophy-focused training, you will lift heavier weight for lower repetitions or perform more dynamic, explosive movements that will fatigue the target muscles faster. Think of running a sprint rather than a marathon. If your goal is to add mass or enlarge your glutes, this training measure may be right for you.

The workouts in this chapter combine exercises performed front to back, side to side, and in rotation. These exercises are presented and explained in part III of this book. Revisit part III for exercise descriptions and cueing; page numbers for the exercises are included with the workouts. Here in chapter 10 are options for sequencing a core workout with hypertrophy focus. You can plug in and play with any of the core exercises presented in this book to create a personal workout; you do not have to stick to only what is presented in this section.

You are strongly encouraged to effectively warm up with the dynamic warm-up program found in chapter 7 before doing any of these workouts. Properly warming up will prepare the body for optimal performance and maximal exercise results. The warm-up is not accounted for in the workout period you see for each workout; your warm-up should take you between 5 and 7 minutes to complete. Also not accounted for is the time you spend cooling down and stretching with stretches found in chapter 8, which should also take between 5 and 7 minutes. The suggested times for your workouts are based on the performance of the average adult exerciser in the United States. The time, sets, repetitions (reps), resistances, and rest periods presented in these workouts are merely suggestions; adjust them to suit your evolving fitness level and ability. You may also choose to do only one or two of the sequences from either of the full workouts in this chapter at the end of a cardio-focused workout (before the cool-down) to add some strength work to your workout.

The following workouts focus on muscular hypertrophy. In other words, they're all about developing mass, lift, and firmness for your butt.

Workout 1: Glutes With Focus on Muscular Hypertrophy

Workout period: 35 to 45 minutes

Number of exercises per workout sequence: 4 or 5 exercises

Sets: 3 to 6 sets for each exercise; 30 to 90 seconds of rest between each set of each exercise

Reps: 6 to 12 reps per set or per your personal preference that can be performed with optimal form. Your last couple of reps should be a challenge or struggle to complete, meaning you can barely do more. If you are able to easily exceed 12 reps, then you probably do not have enough weight or resistance to tax the muscles to build and grow.

Resistance: Moderate to heavy weights that are ideal for muscle growth; in other words, weight that is 65 to 85 percent of your one-repetition maximum (1RM; the maximum weight you can lift for only one repetition with optimal and proper form and alignment)

SAMPLE HYPERTROPHY-FOCUSED GLUTE WORKOUT 1

WORKOUT SEQUENCE 1: COMBO GLUTE EXERCISES		
Exercise	**Exercise photo**	**Page number**
1. Sumo squat		50
2. Hip abduction		81
3. Lateral leg extension		58

(continued)

Sample Hypertrophy-Focused Glute Workout 1 *(continued)*

WORKOUT SEQUENCE 1: COMBO GLUTE EXERCISES *(continued)*		
Exercise	**Exercise photo**	**Page number**
4. Kneeling hip thruster		84
5. Bridge with knee abduction		86

WORKOUT SEQUENCE 2: STANDING GLUTE EXERCISES		
Exercise	**Exercise photo**	**Page number**
1. Squat tapback		42
2. Sumo deadlift		48
3. Standing leg raise		56
4. Pistol squat		54

WORKOUT SEQUENCE 2: STANDING GLUTE EXERCISES *(continued)*		
Exercise	**Exercise photo**	**Page number**
5. Lateral lunge		52

WORKOUT SEQUENCE 3: FLOOR GLUTE EXERCISES		
Exercise	**Exercise photo**	**Page number**
1. Single-leg bridge		90
2. Clam		100
3. Donkey kick		94
4. Seal heel clap		102
5. Butterfly hip lift		92

(continued)

Sample Hypertrophy-Focused Glute Workout 1 *(continued)*

WORKOUT SEQUENCE 4: SEATED, SUPINE, AND KNEELING EXERCISES		
Exercise	**Exercise photo**	**Page number**
1. Incline glute bridge		78
2. Kneeling kickback		82
3. Fire hydrant		88
4. Decline hip bridge		80
5. Hip abduction		81

Workout 2: Glutes With Focus on Muscular Hypertrophy

Workout period: 35 to 45 minutes

Number of exercises per workout sequence: 4 or 5 exercises

Sets: 3 to 6 sets for each exercise; 30 to 90 seconds of rest between each set of each exercise

Reps: 6 to 12 reps per set or per your personal preference that can be performed with optimal form. Your last couple of reps should be a challenge or struggle to complete, meaning you can barely do more. If you are able to easily exceed 12 reps, then you probably do not have enough weight or resistance to tax the muscles to build and grow.

Resistance: Moderate to heavy weights that are ideal for muscle growth; in other words, weight that is 65 to 85 percent of your one-repetition maximum (1RM; the maximum weight you can lift for only one repetition with optimal and proper form and alignment)

SAMPLE HYPERTROPHY-FOCUSED GLUTE WORKOUT 2

WORKOUT SEQUENCE 1: COMBO GLUTE EXERCISES		
Exercise	**Exercise photo**	**Page number**
1. Squat		40
2. Sumo deadlift		48
3. Kneeling hip thruster		84

(continued)

Sample Hypertrophy-Focused Glute Workout 2 *(continued)*

WORKOUT SEQUENCE 1: COMBO GLUTE EXERCISES *(continued)*		
Exercise	**Exercise photo**	**Page number**
4. Incline glute bridge		78
5. Hip abduction		81

WORKOUT SEQUENCE 2: FLOOR-ONLY GLUTE EXERCISES		
Exercise	**Exercise photo**	**Page number**
1. Decline hip bridge		80
2. Donkey kick		94
3. Lunging hip thruster		160
4. Kneeling kickback		82

WORKOUT SEQUENCE 2: FLOOR-ONLY GLUTE EXERCISES *(continued)*		
Exercise	**Exercise photo**	**Page number**
5. Butterfly hip lift		92

WORKOUT SEQUENCE 3: STANDING-ONLY GLUTE EXERCISES		
Exercise	**Exercise photo**	**Page number**
1. Squat to standing leg raise		40, 56
2. Sumo squat		50
3. Squat tapback		42
4. Pistol squat		54

(continued)

Sample Hypertrophy-Focused Glute Workout 2 *(continued)*

WORKOUT SEQUENCE 4: COMBO CORE EXERCISES		
Exercise	**Exercise photo**	**Page number**
1. Sumo squat to lateral flexion to knee		50, 62
2. Lateral lunge to cross-body knee drive		52, 66
3. Incline glute bridge to windshield wiper		78, 124
4. Extended reverse leg lift to plank saw		98, 126

CHAPTER 11
Core Intensity-Focused Workouts

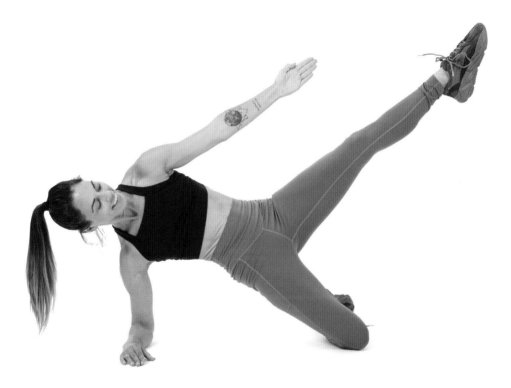

People increase the intensity of their workouts for various reasons. It could be for help in weight loss, to improve athletic performance, or because the body has adapted to previous training styles and needs more progression and challenge. Intensifying an exercise could mean adding more weight, increasing number of repetitions, or moving more explosively. *Intensity* is the level of exerted energy while performing an exercise for a given time frame. To differentiate from training for hypertrophy or endurance, this chapter considers high-intensity interval training (HIIT) as a way of intensifying core training workouts. It is important to maintain proper exercise form and movement quality even with increasing intensity to lessen the risk of injury. Quality movement patterns over quantity and speed will always be a safer and more ideal way of exercising.

The workouts in this chapter combine exercises performed front to back, side to side, and in rotation. These exercises are presented and explained in part III of this book. Revisit part III for exercise descriptions and cueing; page numbers for the exercises are included with the workouts. Presented here in chapter 11 are variations of how each exercise can be paired with another and sequenced for a full workout. You can plug in and play with any of the core exercises presented in this book to create a personal workout; you do not have to stick to only what is presented in this section.

You are strongly encouraged to effectively warm up with the dynamic warm-up program found in chapter 7 before doing any of these workouts. Properly warming up will prepare the body for optimal performance and maximal exercise results. The warm-up is not accounted for in the workout period you see for each workout; your warm-up should take you between 5 and 7 minutes to complete. Also not accounted for is the time you spend cooling down and stretching with stretches found in chapter 8, which should also take between 5 and 7 minutes. The suggested times for your workouts are based on the performance of the average adult exerciser in the United States. The time, sets, repetitions (reps), resistances, and rest periods presented in these workouts are merely suggestions; adjust them to suit your evolving fitness level and ability. You may also choose to do only one or two of the sequences from either of the full workouts in this chapter at the end of a cardio-focused workout (before the cool-down) to add some strength work to your workout.

The following workouts focus on adding intensity to your exercises. In other words, they're about feeling more powerful.

Workout 1: Combination Glute and Ab Workout With Focus on Intensity

Workout period: 30 to 40 minutes

Number of exercises per workout sequence: 3 or 4 exercises per muscle group

Time segments: 30 seconds of work and 30 seconds off, or 45 seconds of work and 15 seconds off; repeat each exercise 3 to 5 times before moving on to the next

Sets: 3 to 5 sets per exercise or paired exercises

Reps: As many reps as possible (AMRAP) done with optimal form. Once you start to lose "good" form, stop the exercise, rest, and then begin again when you're able to move efficiently with optimal form.

Resistance: Body weight or light to moderate weights

SAMPLE INTENSITY-FOCUSED COMBINATION GLUTE AND AB WORKOUT 1

WORKOUT SEQUENCE 1: COMBO GLUTE AND AB EXERCISES		
Exercise	**Exercise photo**	**Page number**
1. Sumo crossbody reach		64
2. Abdominal pushout		114
3. Side plank		122

(continued)

Sample Intensity-Focused Combination Glute and Ab Workout 1 *(continued)*

WORKOUT SEQUENCE 1: COMBO GLUTE AND AB EXERCISES *(continued)*		
Exercise	**Exercise photo**	**Page number**
4. Plank saw		126
5. X sit-up		136
6. Lateral lunge		52
7. Incline glute bridge		78
8. Clam		100
9. Pistol squat		54

WORKOUT SEQUENCE 2: COMBO GLUTE AND AB EXERCISES		
Exercise	**Exercise photo**	**Page number**
1. Sumo squat		50
2. Lunge		44
3. Kneeling hip thruster		84
4. Lateral lunge		52
5. Side-lying clam		158
6. Forward crunch		104

(continued)

Sample Intensity-Focused Combination Glute and Ab Workout 1 *(continued)*

WORKOUT SEQUENCE 2: COMBO GLUTE AND AB EXERCISES *(continued)*		
Exercise	**Exercise photo**	**Page number**
7. Kneeling torso twist		112
8. Sumo lateral crunch		68
9. Plank hip dip		128
WORKOUT SEQUENCE 3: COMBO GLUTE AND AB EXERCISES		
Exercise	**Exercise photo**	**Page number**
1. Pistol squat		54
2. Pilates roll-up		116
3. Decline hip bridge		80

WORKOUT SEQUENCE 3: COMBO GLUTE AND AB EXERCISES *(continued)*		
Exercise	**Exercise photo**	**Page number**
4. Thread the needle		130
5. Fire hydrant		88
6. Abdominal pushout		114
7. Frogger		96
8. Squat tapback		42
9. Side hip tuck		74

Workout 2: Combination Glute and Ab Workout With Focus on Intensity

Workout period: 30 to 40 minutes

Number of exercises per workout sequence: 4 or 5 exercises per muscle group

Time segments: 30 seconds of work and 30 seconds off, or 45 seconds of work and 15 seconds off; repeat each exercise 3 to 5 times before moving on to the next

Sets: 3 to 5 sets per exercise or paired exercises

Reps: As many reps as possible (AMRAP) done with optimal form. Once you start to lose "good" form, stop the exercise, rest, and then begin again when you're able to move efficiently with optimal form.

Resistance: Body weight or light to moderate weights

SAMPLE INTENSITY-FOCUSED COMBINATION GLUTE AND AB WORKOUT 2

WORKOUT SEQUENCE 1: COMBO GLUTE EXERCISES		
Exercise	Exercise photo	Page number
1. Lateral lunge to lateral leg extension		52, 58
2. Pistol squat to single-leg deadlift (deadlift variation)		54, 47
3. Reverse lunge with side reach to lunge		144, 44

WORKOUT SEQUENCE 1: COMBO GLUTE EXERCISES *(continued)*		
Exercise	**Exercise photo**	**Page number**
4. Incline glute bridge to side-lying leg lift (side plank variation)		78, 123
5. Hip abduction		81

WORKOUT SEQUENCE 2: FLOOR-ONLY GLUTE EXERCISES		
Exercise	**Exercise photo**	**Page number**
1. Decline hip bridge to fire hydrant		80, 88
2. Butterfly hip lift to clam		92, 100
3. Frogger		96

(continued)

Sample Intensity-Focused Combination Glute and Ab Workout 2 *(continued)*

WORKOUT SEQUENCE 2: FLOOR-ONLY GLUTE EXERCISES *(continued)*		
Exercise	**Exercise photo**	**Page number**
4. Extended reverse leg lift to seal heel clap		98, 102
WORKOUT SEQUENCE 3: STANDING-ONLY GLUTE EXERCISES		
Exercise	**Exercise photo**	**Page number**
1. Single-leg deadlift (deadlift variation) to pistol squat		47, 54
2. Sumo squat		50
3. Lateral lunge		52
4. Squat		40

WORKOUT SEQUENCE 4: COMBO AB EXERCISES		
Exercise	**Exercise photo**	**Page number**
1. Pilates roll-up to side plank		116, 122
2. K-crunch to thread the needle		110, 130
3. Sumo lateral crunch		68
4. Forward flexion to knee to lateral flexion to knee		60, 62

REFERENCES

CHAPTER 2

Ikeda, D., and S.M. McGill. 2012. "Can Altering Motions, Postures and Loads Provide Immediate Low Back Pain Relief: A Study of 4 Cases Investigating Spine Load, Posture and Stability." *Spine* 37 (23): E1469-75.

Kim, T.W., and Y.W. Kim. 2015. "Effects of Abdominal Drawing-in During Prone Hip Extension on the Muscle Activities of the Hamstring, Gluteus Maximus, and Lumbar Erector Spinae in Subjects With Lumbar Hyperlordosis." *Journal of Physical Therapy Science* 27 (2): 383-86.

McGill, S.M. 2016. *Low Back Disorders: Evidence-Based Prevention and Rehabilitation.* Champaign, IL: Human Kinetics.

ABOUT THE AUTHOR

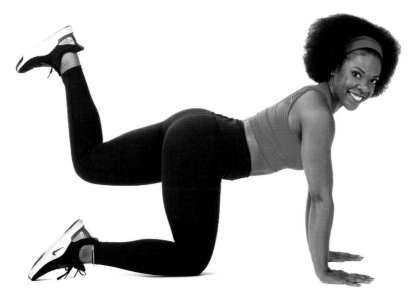

Kia Williams, MBA, MS, RYT 200, is a global presenter, program specialist, business leader, and podcast and web-series host. She was awarded the IDEA Fitness Instructor of the Year in 2022.

An ACE-certified group fitness instructor, Williams (@kiawilliams.fitness) is recognized for her ability to incorporate innovative and progressive exercise techniques that result in enhanced functional fitness, optimal physique, and fun workouts. She has been certified and licensed to teach over a dozen fitness formats and is actively creating content and new formats for children and adults.

Williams has managed several fitness and wellness programs and facilities and uses her transferable professional experience to mentor professionals, champion groundbreaking ideas, support multicultural engagement, and make fitness accessible, inclusive, and feasible for the masses. Kia has a love for all health and wellness categories. Overall, Kia is committed to helping others live a creative, sustainable, gratifying, and healthy lifestyle.

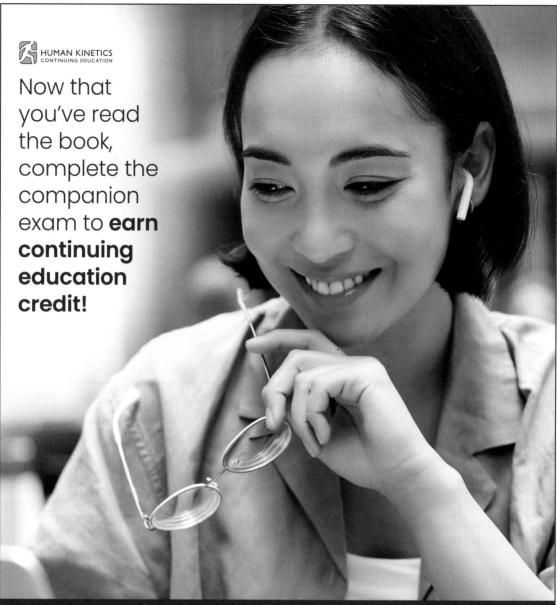
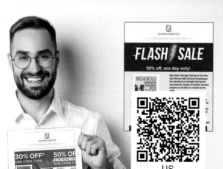